Fasting to Freedom
THE GIFT OF FASTING

CHANTEL RAY

WESTBOW
PRESS®
A DIVISION OF THOMAS NELSON
& ZONDERVAN

This book is a work of non-fiction. Unless otherwise noted, the author and the publisher make no explicit guarantees as to the accuracy of the information contained in this book and in some cases, names of people and places have been altered to protect their privacy.

WestBow Press books may be ordered through booksellers or by contacting:

WestBow Press
A Division of Thomas Nelson & Zondervan
1663 Liberty Drive
Bloomington, IN 47403
www.westbowpress.com
1 (866) 928-1240

Scripture quotations marked (NIV) are taken from the Holy Bible, New International Version®, NIV®. Copyright © 1973, 1978, 1984, 2011 by Biblica, Inc.™ Used by permission of Zondervan. All rights reserved worldwide. www.zondervan.com The "NIV" and "New International Version" are trademarks registered in the United States Patent and Trademark Office by Biblica, Inc.™

Scripture quotations marked (NKJV) taken from the New King James Version®. Copyright © 1982 by Thomas Nelson. Used by permission. All rights reserved.

Scripture quotations marked (NLT) are taken from the Holy Bible, New Living Translation, copyright ©1996, 2004, 2015 by Tyndale House Foundation. Used by permission of Tyndale House Publishers, Inc., Carol Stream, Illinois 60188. All rights reserved.

Scripture quotations marked (AMPC) taken from the Amplified® Bible, Copyright © 1954, 1958, 1962, 1964, 1965, 1987 by The Lockman Foundation Used by permission. www.Lockman.org

ISBN: 978-1-9736-6851-0 (sc)
ISBN: 978-1-9736-6850-3 (e)

Library of Congress Control Number: 2019908969

Print information available on the last page.

WestBow Press rev. date: 08/20/2019

PART 1

Introduction

I spent most of my 20's and 30's feeling defeated, like I was always going to be a slave to food and it would forever have a tight grip on me. I lacked clarity and faced uncertainty and doubt when it came to important decisions. Although I ran a successful real estate business, I didn't feel my impact was reaching its full potential. My health, specifically my thyroid and autoimmune disorders, were just a mess. I was waiting for breakthroughs from God that never seemed to come.

And then, I heard a sermon about fasting and decided to give it a try.

I attended church for my entire adult life without ever hearing a single word about fasting.

What did I have to lose?

Once I began fasting, I started seeing breakthroughs that were happening in my life, so I wanted to fast more and more. I started fasting for one day, which turned into two days, then three days, and so on, working my way up to a 21 day fast!

Before you stop reading this book because you think I am going to ask you to do a 21 day fast, just hear me out!

The bottom line is this: I got really tired of seeing Christians walk around defeated like I used to be, so I had to write this book. I wrote this book because there are so many Christians living in bondage to sin just like I was. Sin that grabs you and won't let go. I call this an enslaving sin, and I talk about it a lot in my book. Maybe you struggle with lust, gossip, greed, alcohol or drug addiction, just to name a few. My enslaving sin was my addiction to food.

I am going to lay out six main reasons why you should fast, and for me, the biggest of them is

> "To loose the chains of injustice and untie the cords
>
> of the yoke, to set the oppressed free and break
>
> every yoke" Isaiah 58:6 (NIV)

In this book I am going to talk about how I felt physically, spiritually, and emotionally during my fasts, so you can hear my experiences. You'll be able to learn from both my experiences and the experiences of some of my friends who did it with me. We are going to talk about bondages and strongholds that were in my life that I was able to defeat through fasting. I will share the rewards I have seen from fasting and the lessons I've learned, and how it has changed my personal walk and brought me into a closer relationship with God. Finally, and most importantly, we are going to talk about what the Bible says about fasting. You are going to learn really practical tips and tricks about how it sharpens your mental processes and can heal your body.

We are going to talk about the fact that fasting is hard! The longest fast that I did was for 21 days. Seven days with coffee and tea only, another seven days with bone broth and smoothies, and the final seven days adding whole fruits and vegetables. It was honestly the longest 21 days of my life. There were days where I was very hangry. My thyroid and autoimmune issues have been an ongoing struggle, and on these ongoing fasts, they present an extra set of challenges.

Despite how hard it is, in the last year I've done at least one hundred 24 hour fasts, twenty four 2 day fasts, ten 3 day fasts, two 5 day fasts, one 8 day fast, and one 21 day fast.

You may be reading this the same way I would have read it a few years ago and thinking "Wow, this chick is crazy, I feel sick when I skip breakfast! Why would I ever consider going days without food?" Just keep reading.

Here are a couple of testimonies from my friends:

> "Through fasting, things are revealed to me that I would never have paid attention to before or would have missed because I was so busy. It brings me closer to God because I am more cognizant and

deliberate in my time with him. I have been praying for my husband to accept Christ for years, and although he still hasn't, I can see God beginning to work in his heart and soften it." - Heather

"When I am fasting, my worship with God is sweeter. My prayers are deeper and more meaningful. I find myself praying for things I would never have thought of on my own."- Ally

"I struggle with depression, and, quite unexpectedly, fasting has really helped me with that. I think that a lot of depression and anxiety come from a feeling of being out of control, and fasting has helped me take back the control that food had over me. It's better than any anti-depressant, and the side effects are much better!"- Andrea

Through this book, you'll discover how you can see supernatural healing in your body; learn how to discern God's still, small whisper to guide you and help you make decisions; utilize God's power to overcome difficult times and receive breakthroughs when you are stuck; experience God's provision in an area that is now lacking; rise up against haters with God's protection; and finally, once and for all, taste victory over a nagging area of sin in your life.

Chapter 1
WHAT IS FASTING ?

I compare the power of fasting to scuba diving. I live in Virginia Beach, and if you stand on the shore and look at the water, it's brownish-black and hard to see beneath the surface. But when you dive deep beneath the surface, everything changes. Although I have never been scuba diving, I've been snuba diving and the difference is that you don't go down quite as deep. Snuba diving is a combination of snorkeling and scuba diving. It doesn't require an air tank underwater, only a tank that sits above the water. With snuba diving you can breathe underwater without coming up for air and you don't have the weight of the scuba diving equipment. You're just connected by like a 20- foot air hose and it follows your every move and allows you to swim around. Anyways, every time I go snuba diving I find hidden treasures that I've never been able to see before. There are so many rare fish, animals, and plants that are in the ocean that you never even knew about! I feel like the fish whisperer, because they come so close to me and I can see all these different details in the fish. There are things that you see that you would never be able to imagine. You get to see the beautiful tropical fish in the coral reefs, and you can see the shells and all the different type of amazing fish. Everything comes alive! Fasting does that for your spirit. Your body is hungry when you fast, but your spirit is sharp and everything comes into focus.

Another thing that fasting does is allow you to "tune in" to God's voice in your Christian walk. The radio station KLOVE on 90.7 is my favorite radio station to listen to in Virginia Beach. If I drive to Richmond to visit my sister; however, I can't hear the station anymore. All I get is static. Doesn't that happen to us sometimes as Christians? We get busy and preoccupied with life and we rarely slow down to hear God's voice. Fasting is like putting spiritual antennas on your ears - you're tuned in to God's station and you can hear clearly.

I own a real estate company, and we do a lot of radio ads. I visit the stations all of the time and record commercials most popular, well-loved DJ's. One of my favorite DJ's, Jimmy Ray Dunn, even left his station to join my real estate company! I am a big fan of radio! God is always communicating with us, but we need to make sure that we are tuned in to his frequency.

We advertise locally on about 10 to 12 different radio stations, and when we get the bills for our ads in the mail they won't say "94.9 the Point," which is the advertised name on the radio station. The bill will say something like WPTE. So, then my accounting director has to go back and see which station is WPTE. If you pay attention, most radio stations have a four letter identification, and it usually starts with a W or a K, like WTKR which is another popular news station that we have here, and of course, KLOVE my favorite station. When we are fasting, it helps us tune into WGOD radio and get on his frequency so that we can hear from Him!

Think about a grape, it's a pretty basic, inexpensive fruit that you can buy just about anywhere. There's not much that you can do with grapes to make them more potent and more powerful than to crush them under your feet to make wine. Now wine is a powerful, potent substance that can be very expensive and valuable. Think about fasting as a means of crushing our sins and our worldly desires and putting our flesh under direct pressure to turn us into something more powerful, more potent than we could ever imagine!

So, what is fasting? Fasting, by definition, is abstaining from food or drink for a period of time. The term "fast" in the Bible comes from the Hebrew word "tsum" literally meaning to "cover the mouth (Strong's Hebrew). In the Greek language, it's "néstis". It combines né- (meaning not) and esthió (meaning to eat) (Strong's Greek). This is the kind of fasting we will talk about in this study. We're not fasting social media or television. We're fasting in the true Biblical sense and that is to not eat.

There are many different fasting practices, including intermittent fasting, which I used to lose 40 pounds. I wrote a book about it called *Waist Away: The Chantel Ray Way*. This book, however, is about **Biblical fasting** and its ability to break chains in your life. Through Biblical fasting, I broke the stronghold of my food addiction, cured my body of many different illnesses, got through difficult times, improved my ability to hear from God, gained clarity when making major decisions, and developed a closer relationship with God. Biblical fasting is not just about going without food for a certain amount of time. **Biblical fasting is about going without food in order to grow closer to God.**

Many different religions have some form of fasting in them. I have Hindu neighbors who fast because they feel it creates a tighter union with God. I have Buddhist friends who fast to be closer to God. My father's family is Muslim and they fast in the daylight hours during the month of Ramadan to get blessings, create self-discipline, and purify their bodies. The fasting we discuss in this book is based on Christian Biblical principles. However, if you're of a different religion, the principles still work.

I believe that fasting needs to be a part of your Christian practice, and the Bible backs me up on this. Fasting is mentioned over 77 times in Scripture. In Matthew 6, Jesus teaches us about three Christian disciplines: praying, giving and fasting.

Matthew 6:2 (NIV)

[2] "So when you give to the needy …

Matthew 6:5 (NIV)

[5] "And when you pray …

Matthew 6:16 (NIV)

[16] "When you fast …

WHEN you give …

WHEN you pray …

WHEN you fast …

Jesus expected us to do all of these things and we should give as much attention to fasting as we do to praying and giving. I think the reason many Christians don't fast is because it's not talked about very much in the modern church. I had never heard a sermon on fasting for the first 20 years of my Christian life! Here's what Jesus had to say about fasting:

Matthew 6:16-18 (NIV)

16 "When you fast, do not look somber as the hypocrites do, for they disfigure their faces to show others they are fasting. Truly I tell you, they have received their reward in full. 17 But when you fast, put oil on your head and wash your face, 18 so that it will not be obvious to others that you are fasting, but only to your Father, who is unseen; and your Father, who sees what is done in secret, will reward you.

Jesus doesn't say how often or how long we should fast - that's between you and God. You don't need to tell everyone you're on a fast, but you can share it with your spiritual partner. I absolutely believe that you should fast with friends, if you can. Fasting is not easy, so it's very important to have people around you that can encourage, strengthen, and pray with you.

I believe that one of the greatest appetites human beings have is for food. It's a strong, natural desire that we deny when we fast. We are activating power in our lives when we do this by getting closer to God. **I don't believe that God is growing closer to us when we fast. I believe that we are growing closer to God when we fast.**

Luke 5:33-35 (NIV)

33 They said to him, "John's disciples often fast and pray, and so do the disciples of the Pharisees, but yours go on eating and drinking."

34 Jesus answered, "Can you make the friends of the bridegroom fast while he is with them? 35 But the time will come when the bridegroom will be taken from them; in those days they will fast."

In this passage, the Pharisees criticized the disciples for not fasting, but Jesus explained they would fast when they needed to: after He was gone. He basically said, "Look, I'm with these guys right now. They don't need to fast because they're right next to me! After I'm gone, they'll fast to get closer to me and hear from me." Isn't that a powerful passage? We learn from these scriptures why we fast and that, once again, Jesus expects us to fast. In my opinion, fasting is not an option. It is essential.

1 Peter 2:21 (NIV)

21 To this you were called, because Christ suffered for you, leaving you an example, that you should follow in his steps.

Since we're called to follow Christ's example, our question should be, "Did Jesus fast?"

HE DID!

Matthew 4:1-2 (NIV)

⁴ Then Jesus was led by the Spirit into the wilderness to be tempted by the devil. ⁵After fasting forty days and forty nights, he was hungry.

Jesus did the ultimate fast! I'm not suggesting you fast for 40 days, but what a serious example! I teach more about overeating, the pull of food, and breaking the stronghold of food in my book, *Waist Away: The Chantel Ray Way.* I encourage you to read it if you're someone who struggles with weight loss, food addiction, or dieting. Fasting is not just a physical discipline. Fasting is you filling up your spiritual tank.

Psalm 34:8 (NIV)

⁸ Taste and see that the Lord is good; blessed is the one who takes refuge in him.

Fasting is telling God that you hunger for more of His presence, wisdom, and clarity in your life. Personally, overeating is the sin that I struggle with most. Some of you have been battling the same enslaving sin over and over again. You've tried to get out of bondage but you keep coming back to it over and over. It's going to take more than just praying about it to get rid of that sin in your life.

I've talked to a lot of people about fasting and here are some of the reasons they told me they don't do it:

- I have really low blood sugar. It doesn't have anything to do with my faith, it's just that my body won't allow me to not eat every couple of hours

- What does me not eating have to do with growing closer to God?

- I've never even heard of spiritual fasting, they don't talk about it at my church

- I won't be able to function without food, I won't be able to go to work and be productive in my day-to-day activities

- If I am hungry, it will actually distract me from growing closer to God because all I will be able to think about is food

- I don't have anyone who is interested in fasting with me, and I can't do it alone

- I have a busy social life, with parties and work lunches, and people will look at me funny if I am not eating.

Most of these are logical excuses, but they are just that, excuses. Let's break them down one by one. First, the blood sugar. I have low blood sugar myself! The crazy thing about fasting is that is has actually helped regulate my blood sugar. The more fasting I have done, the more stable my blood sugar has become. There is science behind fasting as it relates to blood sugar.

What does not eating have to do with growing closer to God? As you'll see in this book, fasting is all over the Bible, mentioned over 70 times! If Moses, Elijah, David, and even Jesus himself fasted, why would we somehow be above it? They don't talk about fasting at your church? Find a new church. Just kidding!

As I mentioned, I didn't hear about fasting at church for years! There are some great resources online, sermons and podcasts. I am praying this book is a great resource to get you started!

We live in the information age, and everything we want to learn and discover is at our finger tips. If you don't think you will be able to function without food, I dare you to try! I run a multi-million dollar real estate company with over 200 employees; to say we are busy is an understatement! But in time, I saw that the clarity and focus I gain from fasting has actually helped my business immensely, and over time, has even made me more productive. Even on the days that I may be struggling on a fast and don't feel as productive, I've noticed that my coworkers seem to have an extra boost of energy. They will come to me and say, "Oh my goodness, you will never believe, I was able to do A, B, C, and D today!"

Do you think that you will not grow closer to God because you will be too obsessed thinking about food? You might have a similar stronghold to food in your life that I did and may need to reevaluate your relationship with food all together. Fasting has truly freed me from the bondage I experienced with food for most of my life. Don't have any friends that want to fast with you? Find some new friends. Just kidding! When I first started fasting, I was doing it all alone. As soon as my friends started seeing my breakthroughs and the level of intimacy with God I was experiencing, they wanted in on it too. Not all of my friends fast, but I have a couple of close friends who do it with me. Pray for friends like these! Are you worried about how fasting will interfere with your social life? I have been to hundreds of functions while I've been fasting, and I guarantee you that no one cares what I am eating! They are more concerned about what they are eating! The whole goal in going out to eat or to a function with a group of people is to bond, socialize, network and connect. Not eating doesn't get in the way of the goal. You'll see lots of examples of this in the book, even one story in which I went to one of the nicest restaurants in New York City with a colleague who was paying the bill and I didn't eat at all. And still had a great time!

It boils down to this- the main reason people don't fast is because it's hard! At no point do I want you to think that fasting will be easy. But nothing good in life comes easily. If you want a good marriage, it's going to require hard work. If you want a successful career, it's going to require hard work. Raising Godly children is definitely hard. Many of you struggle with your weight and will agree that maintaining a healthy, fit body is hard. You get the point! We live in a world of short cuts, magic pills and secret sauces. Everyone I know who is successful at anything has had trials, struggles, naysayers, and setbacks. But they didn't give up and you shouldn't either. I've done a ton of fasting, and it still isn't easy for me! But you need to press on, hang in there, and just keep moving. Anything worthwhile is going to be hard, but worth it.

If I said to you, "I want you to spend five minutes in prayer," that may feel like a long time, but it's doable. Attending church for an hour or two each week may seem like a sacrifice to some, but it's not that much in the scheme of week. Even if you add in an hour of attending small group, it's a sacrifice, but not a stretch. Fasting is a real stretch! Not eating for one day, two days, three days- that is a real stretch of faith. I know a lot of really strong Christians who still think they need to eat every two hours. They can be extremely disciplined in every area of their spiritual walk but refuse to submit to this one discipline. I have a close family member that is this way. She is sold out for God, completely submitted, but she refuses to fast. She buys into the lies from the devil that her blood sugar won't allow for fasting. She literally eats the moment she wakes up every day and continues to eat every two hours, even if it's something like almonds.

I believe that these Christians, like my family member, who refuse to fast are really missing out on all that God has for them.

Fasting has truly changed my life, and I am praying that through this book, it will change yours as well.

Chapter 2

WHY SHOULD I FAST?

In this book, we will learn how to use the power of Biblical fasting to heal our bodies and hear from God, overcome adversity, receive provision and protection from God, and break free from enslaving sins. I like to use the acronym of HOPE when it comes to fasting. HOPE can outline reasons that we should choose to fast:

<u>HOPE</u>

Reasons We Fast (Insert Image):

H- Heal and Hear

O- Overcome Difficult Times

P- Provision and Protection

E- Enslaving Sins

There is a passage that I love in Isaiah, and when I was reading it, I realized that it covers every single one of these letters in the acronym.

"⁵Is not this the kind of fasting I have chosen:

to loose the chains of injustice

and untie the cords of the yoke,

to set the oppressed free

and break every yoke?

[7] Is it not to share your food with the hungry

and to provide the poor wanderer with shelter—

when you see the naked, to clothe them,

and not to turn away from your own flesh and blood?

[8] Then your light will break forth like the dawn,

and your healing will quickly appear;

then your righteousness will go before you,

and the glory of the LORD will be your rear guard.

[9] Then you will call, and the LORD will answer;

you will cry for help, and he will say: Here am I.

"If you do away with the yoke of oppression,

with the pointing finger and malicious talk,

[10] and if you spend yourselves in behalf of the hungry

and satisfy the needs of the oppressed,

then your light will rise in the darkness,

and your night will become like the noonday.

[11] The LORD will guide you always;

he will satisfy your needs in a sun-scorched land

and will strengthen your frame.

You will be like a well-watered garden,

like a spring whose waters never fail.

¹² Your people will rebuild the ancient ruins

and will raise up the age-old foundations;

you will be called Repairer of Broken Walls,

Restorer of Streets with Dwellings. Isaiah 58:5-12 (NIV)

HOPE

H- Heal and Hear

Heal Isaiah 58:8 (NIV)

⁸Then your light will break forth like the dawn,

and your healing will quickly appear

Hear Isaiah 58:9 (NIV)

⁹you will call, and the LORD will answer

O- Overcome Difficult Times Isaiah 58:10 (NIV)

¹⁰you will find your joy in the LORD

your light will rise in the darkness,

and your night will become like the noonday

P- Provision and Protection

Provision Isaiah 58:11 (NIV)

¹¹The LORD will guide you always;

he will satisfy your needs in a sun-scorched land

and will strengthen your frame.

Protection Isaiah 58:8 (NIV)

[8]then your righteousness will go before you,

and the glory of the LORD will be your rear guard.

E- Enslaving Sins Isaiah 58:6 (NIV)

[6]to loose the chains of injustice

and untie the cords of the yoke,

to set the oppressed free

and break every yoke?

You might be looking at this acronym and saying "Wow, I am not really struggling with any of these things right now," I guess I don't need to fast.

I have found that one of the major reasons why Christians have stopped fasting is because a lot of the time they may find that they don't have that much to worry about. They may not have trouble paying the bills or may not have trouble with health, so they find themselves wondering why they should fast if everything is going okay. When people are in this mindset, and something bad happens in their lives, they may wonder why they didn't fast. But, maybe they aren't hearing from God in a really vivid way or don't have clarity on the decisions they are making. So, they then find themselves in a pickle and wonder why they didn't fast about a decision in the first place. A lot of the time, I hear people saying that they don't know what God wants them to do. They feel like God has let them down and that He's not there for them.

When we're not fasting, or hearing from Him, or allowing Him to take our burdens from us, we may not realize that we would be able to experience a whole new level with God through fasting. We have gotten to a place where it is difficult to fast, so it is essential that you find yourself in a place where you really want to take your walk with God to the next level. You have to be able to give up the comfort of where you are. As much as we may not like to admit it, food is comforting. With fasting, it does have a level of pain when this is taken away. When you're fasting, you have to be willing to say, "I'm okay with the level of pain I'm in right now. My hunger in wanting to grow in my walk with God is more than this small pain of not being able to eat." Feeling this pain is natural, though. We all are selfish and Proverbs 16:26 (NIV) highlights this:

Proverbs 16:26 (NIV) [26]"The appetite of laborers work for them; their hunger drives them on"

Sometimes when we fast, we're fasting for the wrong motives like wanting to lose weight or fasting because we want something from God and think that if we fast then He will reward us with what we want Him to do. Prayer and fasting does take effort, which is basically the number one reason why Christians don't pray and fast. It just doesn't rate high on their priority list. It ends up that you put something else ahead of praying and fasting. If you choose not to fast because you have to work or are already going to the gym, you are making whatever it is a higher priority.

Your flesh and your body are not going to want you to fast. You're going to constantly make excuses. You may think that now isn't the best time to do this or that you may offend other members of your family because they're making a big meal for you. The list can go on and on. The devil is going to try to give you every possible excuse that he can. That is why you have to make sure that you make the commitment. Start small and then move forward. There's a passage in Psalms that I want to share in regards to this:

Psalm 109:24 (NIV)

"My knees are weak from fasting and my body is

thin and gaunt."

In this passage, David is explaining how he was feeling physically, however he goes on to say how strong his spirit had become because of it. Fasting is not easy and does take a physical toll on your body. What we tend to underestimate is how much it can help our spirits grow. It seems like most people fast when there is a problem or when they want to hear from God. This seems to be the only time we can convince ourselves to do it. I think fasting builds up your faith and really helps you when you are both in crisis or when you need to be prepared for crisis. Fasting can prepare you to share your faith with others and show how seriously you take God's word.

1 Corinthians 9:27 (NIV)

"No, I strike a blow to my body and make it my slave

so that after I have preached to others, I myself will

not be disqualified for the prize."

I always feel like there is usually one reason in the HOPE acronym that you are led to fast or make that choice. Even if your fasting is not for a material thing but is just to get closer to God, it is still good to have one clearly defined prayer request for that fast.

Usually, when I do a fast, there are 3-4 items, typically three is the number of the things I am praying for, and usually I am doing the fast with two other people, so I will say, "What are we praying for?" If you don't have focused requests, you won't have focused thanks to give God at the end.

On a recent extended fast, one of my friends wanted to pray for a Godly husband, and the other friend is married but her husband doesn't know Christ, so she wants to pray for him to come to the Lord. For me, I was really fasting to pray for my health and thyroid issues, my physical health.

At the end of the fast, I still had thyroid issues, my one friend was still single, and my other friend's husband hadn't accepted Christ. And this is okay! You need to make sure that you don't feel the fast is a waste if you don't see an answer to your prayer requests immediately. Sometimes you will not see a result right away. It would be easy for my friend who was praying for a Godly husband to say "Hey, I just fasted for two days and I don't even have a date!" But you can't give up.

Fasting is really hard, and you need specific, important reasons to be doing it, so that the hope of your reward outweighs the hardship of your sacrifice.

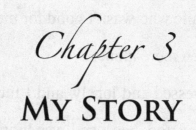

Chapter 3
MY STORY

Before we go any further, I want to tell you a little more about my experience with fasting, and the enslaving sin that I have struggled with for most of my adult life. I have a whole chapter later in the book about Enslaving Sins, but for now I will just say that enslaving sins are those pesky, stubborn sins that you just can't shake no matter how hard you try.

I struggled with food my entire life. I unknowingly used food emotionally from the time I was about 12 or 13-years-old. At the time, I didn't know anything about the term "emotional eating," but I was definitely doing my fair share of it! Food comforted me.

I reached my lowest point in college. I was a math major, and I was completely out of my league. In high school, even though I never studied, I was great at math. However, once we stopped working with straight up numbers in my third year of college, I realized I wasn't as naturally smart at math as I had been before and that it just wasn't easy anymore. I was also used to having a ton of friends growing up, but once I got to college, I only had a few. I felt like I was hanging out with nothing but math nerds from my class and I felt lonely.

I even dated a guy for a while who wasn't good for me to fill that void, and that breakup left me feeling even more alone.

I was completely stressed and lonely, and I literally made food my new best friend. It was my enemy, too, because I was living on a tiny budget. When my clothes stopped fitting, I didn't have money to buy new ones. My pattern was to binge and then starve, binge again and start a new diet, and then fail. Eventually, I started throwing up. Instead of running to God, I ran to food to handle all of the pressure I was under.

Food has had a strong hold on people since Adam and Eve's time. Even they were not free from its grip! Let's look at their story to begin, and dissect how we as humans, and Christians, see food. Why has food become such an idol in our lives? It has been this way since the very beginning.

Genesis 2:16-17 (NIV)

16 And the Lord God commanded the man, "You are free to eat from any tree in the garden; 17 but you must not eat from the tree of the knowledge of good and evil, for when you eat from it you will certainly die."

Genesis 3:1-7 (NIV)

1Now the serpent was more crafty than any of the wild animals the Lord God had made. He said to the woman, "Did God really say, 'You must not eat from any tree in the garden'?"

² The woman said to the serpent, "We may eat fruit from the trees in the garden, ³but God did say, 'You must not eat fruit from the tree that is in the middle of the garden, and you must not touch it, or you will die.'"

⁴ "You will not certainly die," the serpent said to the woman. ⁵ "For God knows that when you eat from it your eyes will be opened, and you will be like God, knowing good and evil."

⁶ When the woman saw that the fruit of the tree was good for food and pleasing to the eye, and also desirable for gaining wisdom, she took some and ate it. She also gave some to her husband, who was with her, and he ate it. ⁷Then the eyes of both of them were opened, and they realized they were naked; so, they sewed fig leaves together and made coverings for themselves.

Adam and Eve went from perfection and enjoying God's presence to nakedness, shame, and passing the blame with just one bite of fruit. Their minds and stomachs were temporarily satisfied, but they suffered massive consequences. That same thing happens to us when we overeat; we satisfy our appetites, but we suffer so many consequences.

Food is so important to us that the love of food has invaded every part of our culture. I watched a TV show recently in which a guy decided to call off his wedding when he found out that his fiancé had deceived him into thinking she could cook when she couldn't. I guess her other traits (personality, character, spirituality, etc.) didn't matter as much to him. Food has become like an idol to us. Today, there are countless people dealing with anxiety and depression who turn to food for comfort. They use food to comfort and relax themselves. For these people, food has become something they can't even think about living without. If you ever try to take away their food, it's like taking away their joy.

This is true for a lot of people, including many Christians. Because, in the Christian world, food is the most acceptable idol. It's one of the most powerful gods I see reigning in Christian lives. Notice how the Christian gatherings that draw the most attendance all revolve around food, whether they are BBQs, picnics, or banquets. Nowadays, you have to promise a huge and lavish spread to guarantee people will show up. I remember we spent thousands of dollars on food for my first book launch that drew 350 people. Ironically, the book was about fasting for weight loss! Whatever the event, food has to be front and center in your advertising if you want to draw a crowd. Have you ever thought about that?

In the Church, we laugh about our love affair with food, but it's not funny at all. Paul said in Philippians that by making our bellies our god, we've made ourselves enemies of the cross.

Philippians 3:17-19 (NIV)

[17] Join together in following my example, brothers and sisters, and just as you have us as a model,

keep your eyes on those who live as we do. [18] For, as I have often told you before and now tell you again even with tears, many live as enemies of the cross of Christ. [19] Their destiny is destruction, their god is their stomach, and their glory is in their shame. Their mind is set on earthly things.

See, food is not a very good god because it can only satisfy you temporarily. That's why using food for anything other than fuel is a disaster waiting to happen

John 6:27 (NIV)

[27] Do not work for food that spoils, but for food that endures to eternal life, which the Son of Man will give you. For on him God the Father has placed his seal of approval."

The Bible doesn't play when it comes to overeating or gluttony, this is one verse that I have memorized and try to quote when I am tempted to overeat:

Proverbs 23:1-2 (NIV)

[1] When you sit to dine with a ruler, note well what is before you, [2] and put a knife to your throat if you are given to gluttony.

We know this scripture isn't encouraging you to commit suicide. It's telling you to curb your appetite! You must be in control instead of your stomach. Why?

Proverbs 23:21 (NIV)

²¹ for drunkards and gluttons become poor, and drowsiness clothes them in rags.

See how the Bible puts gluttons (overeaters) and drunkards in the same class? We don't do that today in the Church. We have a double standard. We would never allow a pastor to lead a church if he was a drunkard, but we don't mind gluttony one bit.

So that's my struggle, with food and my flesh. I am sure that you have struggles of your own, and, like me, you may feel like they will haunt you forever. I want to talk about the idea of HOPE before we move on, and why it was so important for me to incorporate this acronym in the book.

Proverbs 13:12 (NIV)

¹² Hope deferred makes the heart sick, but a longing fulfilled is a tree of life.

If you long for something over and over again and don't get what you want, you start to feel discouraged and want to give up and it makes your heart sick. But when you get the desire you are hoping for, you feel invigorated and alive, like the tree of life.

We created this acronym HOPE because when you have an issue with any of these things: hearing from God, healing for your body and soul, overcoming different times, lacking provision, seeking protection, and being enslaved by sin, you, literally, can experience symptoms that are similar to depression.

With my food issues and eating, there were times I got to a state of hopelessness and discouragement and felt depressed and frustrated. If you can't make a breakthrough in a particular area, a lot of people just give up.

I truly thought I would be overweight and enslaved to food for the rest of my life. I don't know why, but I have a stronghold in this area. When I feel like I have unrelenting disappointment, which is the same thing as hope deferred, I just want to give up.

But when I started fasting, I noticed that every time I finished a fast I was slowly chiseling away at my stronghold with food and I had more hope. After every fast, I had some hope that food would not forever have a stronghold in my life. Still today, I fast, and I notice the stronghold being chiseled away. And so on. For me, I have to do fasts every week, either for 24 hours, 48 hours, or three days. But, I want you to get rid of the notion that fasting is a one time cure all. It's not; it's a practice.

When you have an area that you can't seem to breakthrough, it's so much easier to just give up in that area. It can end up being the "thorn in your side." You end up giving into it, thinking, "it is what it is."

There are some areas in your life that the battle is going to take a long time. If you've spent 30 years learning how to overeat, learning how not to overeat is not going to be a short battle to win. Every time that you give in to the enemy, he gets stronger. Every time you don't give in, you get stronger. I love to use the story of me smoking cigarettes in the past as an example. When I was younger, in my early twenties, I was smoking cigarettes regularly. Every time I tried to quit, I would fail. When I decided that I was finally going to win, I did. After I went about 30 days without smoking, I knew I had won. You literally couldn't pay me to smoke a cigarette now. However, it was the hardest thing to give up. It takes 30 days of doing the same thing over and over for it to become a habit.

I've struggled with overeating for 20 years. Only after prayer and fasting did I succeed in overcoming this struggle. With my weight loss, I got to a place where I kind of just accepted it. I thought, "I don't curse, I don't smoke, and I don't commit adultery, so I'm not so bad." Everyone has a vice, and unfortunately, I thought that this was mine and that I couldn't really fix it. It was the thorn in my side, and it was my thing that I couldn't quit. I could have stayed in that place, but I realized this problem wasn't something Jesus was going to just take away. So, I had to deal with it.

Some of the other habits I've created for myself include only eating when my stomach growls, eating in a 6 hour window, chewing my food 25-50 times, and having a juice or smoothie instead of a full meal at times. You need to make your set of rules for your own battlefield, whatever that is. Every time you break one of these rules or give in, it becomes easier the next time. Another good analogy of this is to compare it to having sex before marriage. The first time you have sex before marriage, you may find yourself feeling guilty or bad about it.

Then each time after, it can become easier to give in. This is no different than any other rule you've set for yourself. Once you give in, it is hard to stop there. Again, just because it's a long battle doesn't mean it's a losing battle.

I cannot stress this enough. I ask myself questions about this when I don't know how to overcome something or when I'm unsure why it's something I have been struggling with so long and just can't seem to break. It is one of those things where you just have to think, "Okay, even though it's taken me a long time to get here, I know that it's going to be a longer battle and I still have work to do." I find a lot of people who are Christians don't like a long battle and they just give up when things don't seem to go their way immediately. However, the battle is all part of the growth process. Don't give up yet just because it's been a long time. It doesn't have to mean it's going to be a loss.

Here's a story about someone who was desperate for a breakthrough. Let's see what he did first:

Matthew 17:14-15 (NKJV)

[14] And when they had come to the multitude, a man came to Him, kneeling down to Him and saying, [15] "Lord, have mercy on my son, for he is an epileptic and suffers severely; for he often falls into the fire and often into the water.

He came humbly to the Lord begging for mercy. When deciding if fasting is the right decision for you, you should come humbly to God and ask for mercy to help in a problem you can't fix on your own. Let's dig further into the passage by reading it from the Gospel of Mark.

Mark 9:21 (NKJV)

21 So He asked his father, "How long has this been happening to him?"

And he said, "From childhood.

It is so important to remember that these bondages we are dealing with aren't ones of sins and temptations. These are long-standing struggles.

Mark 9:22 (NKJV)

22 And often he has thrown him both into the fire and into the water to destroy him. But if You can do anything, have compassion on us and help us."

Ask God for mercy and to have compassion on you.

Mark 9:24-29 (NKJV)

24 Immediately the father of the child cried out and said with tears, "Lord, I believe; help my unbelief!"

25 When Jesus saw that the people came running together, He rebuked the unclean spirit, saying to it: "Deaf and dumb spirit, I command you, come out of him and enter him no more!" 26 Then *the spirit* cried out, convulsed him greatly,

and came out of him. And he became as one dead, so that many said, "He is dead." [27] But Jesus took him by the hand and lifted him up, and he arose.

[28] And when He had come into the house, His disciples asked Him privately, "Why could we not cast it out?"

[29] So He said to them, "This kind can come out by nothing but prayer and fasting."

Chapter 4
GOD'S REWARDS FOR FASTING

Hebrews 11:6 (NIV)

**⁶ And without faith it is impossible to please God,
because anyone who comes to him must believe that
he exists and that he rewards those who earnestly
seek him.**

I want to share some of the rewards that I have seen people receive as a result of fasting. One of my friends in my Bible study group has a 17-year-old teenager who suffered from really bad acne. He had oozing acne and had tried everything to fix it. I asked him if he would be willing to do a 3-day fast with me because I thought it would make a huge difference. He agreed and I interceded for him in prayer for those three days. Afterward, his face completely changed. I have another friend whose father-in-law was in the hospital and close to death according to the doctors. We fasted and prayed and a day later he went home! They couldn't explain it. It was a miracle.

Another example is a time when we were having a rough couple of months at our real estate company. In our economy we were having a government shutdown, and a ton of people in our area are government employees. In general in our business, January and February are the slowest months of the year for closings. They are very good for getting new business, but because people are winding down in November and December, with the holidays and everything, there is not much on the books to close in January. Usually we make a little profit in January or February, or will at least break even. But this particular January, it was awful. I called some of my friends that are top agents in other areas, and they told me this month was abysmal for them too. We were thinking, "We would lose about 100k in January because it would be such a low month.

My same friends, Ally and Heather, decided to do a spiritual fast with me for three things:

1. Wisdom on a Salesforce decision

2. Heather's husband to accept Christ (I mentioned him earlier, this is ongoing!)

3. Clarity on a decision we needed to make with a manager that wasn't performing up to expectations.

We just decided that we wanted to focus on those things. We weren't necessarily fasting about our bad month of January, there wasn't anything we could do to add closings to the books for February by fasting, and we had already accepted that the 80k-100k was a loss. But as a result of the fasting, God gave us a way to save $30k in one year with our Salesforce licenses. We also got random things in the mail, like a $6,900 check from REIN, which is our local

MLS, which we weren't expecting! We found out that one of our Branch Office Administrators, Morgan, inquired on a high electric bill at her office, and when she called and found out we were over billed, we got a $6,800 check for that! We switched vendor partners, and the new partner, instead of paying us in arrears, like the old partner did, paid us in advance. So, we received an extra $28k that we weren't expecting! Sometimes when you fast, God takes care of things that you weren't even praying for or asking for. He really provided for us in ways we didn't even think to ask, and I believe it was as a result of our fasting and our faith.

Another time He provided in a way we didn't even ask is when we were asking for clarity ways to make our corporate office more profitable. Out of the blue, we had two employees turn in their notices, freeing up thousands and thousands of dollars in payroll. God works in unexpected ways that we don't even ask sometimes!

I think it's really important that you keep your eyes open for these blessings from God. It would have been really easy to chalk these checks up to coincidence, or to totally miss out on noticing what God was doing. But you have to keep your eyes open for his blessings and take the time to give him credit and thank him.

It reminds me of the story of the ten lepers mentioned in Luke 17:11-19 (NIV). Jesus healed ten lepers, and only one turned around to thank Him! I think this parable, whether it says it or not, reminds us that God does so much for us, but we only recognize it one out of ten times. It doesn't say this in the passage per say, but we miss out on recognizing it and thanking him so often!

I want to remind you again that just because you fast doesn't mean that

God is going to answer all of your prayers. It means you will be able to better deal with whatever God has for you. I had a situation on another 3-day fast, which my company put out an ad looking for photographers to work with us. We offered lower than the standard rate and we got some negative responses.

We got some really nasty comments and the post got a lot of attention. I had a good attitude about it, and God brought scriptures to me to handle the situation. It turned out to be a blessing! We recruited five new agents after that and got more photographers than we know what to do with. God was faithful! Some of those comments may have been mean and nasty, but God was faithful through it all. The scriptures below helped me to maintain positivity throughout the situation:

Genesis 50:20 (NIV)

[20] You intended to harm me, but God intended it for good to accomplish what is now being done, the saving of many lives.

Luke 6:26 (NIV)

[26] Woe to you when everyone speaks well of you, for that is how their ancestors treated the false prophets.

Romans 8:28 (NIV)

[28] And we know that in all things God works for the good of those who love him, who have been called according to his purpose.

Most of the people I talk to find the principle of fasting to be overwhelming. The idea of not eating one meal (let alone two meals, or not eating for three days) is too much for them and they push it down into a corner. Fasting isn't easy, but it is very powerful. You need super willpower to fast. The truth is that you can't do it with your own strength. You need God's strength. Because of this, fasting isn't for the weak. It's so important that you really pray about fasting and prepare yourself for it. Even now, I have to prepare my mind every time I fast. Prepare spiritually and ask God if this is the right time and make sure He's going to give you the extra strength you need. You will feel the Holy Spirit tug on your heart. It's an invitation to get to know Him in a powerful way. You'll get the sense that God is telling you that it's time to fast. At that point, decide what kind of fast you will do and how long it will last for.

PART 2

Your Fasting Guide

Chapter 5

PREPARING FOR YOUR FAST

I spent 20 years in church and never heard a sermon on fasting. My first encounter with it was soon after I joined Beach Fellowship in Virginia Beach and Pastor Ray Bjorkman announced a 21-day fast. It was a huge culture shock! The fast - not always 21 days - was something they did every year because Pastor Ray believed corporate fasts were something that God honored and rewarded. Some great miracles took place during that fast, including people being healed of cancer.

Because fasting was completely new to me, it wreaked havoc on my body. It conflicted with the thyroid medication I was on at the time and I felt miserable. Fasting is like exercise. If you've never done it before, YOU HAVE TO START SMALL! Pastor Ray didn't do anything wrong - in fact, he gave everyone the option to do a shorter fast, if you've never fasted before, don't try to do 21 days! It's like running 21 miles when you're not a runner. It's a recipe for disaster. Just like anything in life, preparation is key.

Here are some ways that I prepare for my fasts:

Step One: First, write down a fasting plan. Whether it's one meal a day or a 24-hour fast, if you don't write it down you will struggle to succeed. You need to write down when your fast starts and the hour it's going to end so that you don't forget. Later in this section, I am going to share some example plans to help you get started.

Making a commitment is the first step to being successful with fasting.

Commitment is a big problem for people in every area of life. I get frustrated when I purchase tables to charity events and the people who promised to come and fill those tables don't show up. It's like since they got in for free they don't feel the need to follow through on their promise. I read resumes all the time from people who can't keep a job for longer than 12 months.

Even marriages suffer from lack of commitment in our society. People give up quickly. My first two years of marriage were rough, and I had times of thinking that it wasn't going to work, but I knew I had made a commitment. We're more in love now than when we started and we're better for it. I always recommend that you have a coach to keep you on track. If you want us to help you with fasting, visit chantelraycoaching.com.

For most people, the decision to fast comes from desperation. Desperation pushes you to do things you normally wouldn't do. Haven't you ever heard stories of mothers who stole food just so they could feed their children? Stealing is not something they did because they were thieves at heart. It was an act of desperation.

Luke 8:40-44 (NIV)

40 Now when Jesus returned, a crowd welcomed him, for they were all expecting him. 41 Then a man named Jairus, a synagogue leader, came and fell at Jesus' feet, pleading with him to come to his house 42 because his only daughter, a girl of about twelve, was dying.

As Jesus was on his way, the crowds almost crushed him. 43 And a woman was there who had been subject to bleeding for twelve years, but no one could heal her. 44 She came up behind him and touched the edge of his cloak, and immediately her bleeding stopped.

This woman probably wouldn't have put herself in such a dangerous position if she weren't desperate and determined. She could have been stoned for being outside in her condition, but she was willing to do whatever it took. That determination got her healed. When we're desperate, we need to go to Jesus' feet and fast and pray. Sometimes, it's a long road to healing. It was for me. For most of my life I had an eating addiction that damaged my body. Now, every time I fast, my body gets better and better. I'm not 100%, but I'm getting there! Before you say fasting doesn't work, remember that it's a process. It takes time to heal yourself from this bondage in your life. The woman with the issue of blood was sick for 12 years. Some of you have struggled with some sort of bondage even longer.

It can take time for God to mature your faith. He wants you to have a stubborn faith, so that nothing can shake you. Most of us focus so much on life's curveballs and create resentment toward God. Curveballs are your friend and God uses them for your benefit! Take the passenger seat and let God fly the plane. Trust Him to be bigger than the problem.

Luke 8:49-55 (NIV)

49 While Jesus was still speaking, someone came from the house of Jairus, the synagogue leader. "Your daughter is dead," he said. "Don't bother the teacher anymore."

50 Hearing this, Jesus said to Jairus, "Don't be afraid; just believe, and she will be healed."

51 When he arrived at the house of Jairus, he did not let anyone go in with him except Peter, John and James, and the child's father and mother. 52 Meanwhile, all the people were wailing and mourning for her. "Stop wailing," Jesus said. "She is not dead but asleep."

53 They laughed at him, knowing that she was dead. 54 But he took her by the hand and said, "My child, get up!" 55 Her spirit returned, and at once she stood up. Then Jesus told them to give her something to eat.

Jairus is another portrait of a desperate person. He was a high-ranking official in the synagogue that was run by people who hated Jesus. Going to Him cost Jairus something. It's going to cost you something, too. I have friends who won't fast because it "doesn't work well" for them. Of course it doesn't! Fasting isn't about being comfortable. Only desperate people are interested in this. I got desperate and decided that I didn't want to be sick and in bondage to food anymore. I got desperate enough to make sacrifices and stop making excuses. That's what it takes to be healed. You can't be wishy-washy.

Step Two: Involve your loved ones, or at least make them aware. Sometimes you have to put relationships and entertainment on the back burner. You don't have to RSVP "yes" to every invitation that comes your way. I get invited to parties and fundraisers literally every weekend, but when I'm fasting I have to put them to the side and know how to say "no."

Write down your goals on paper and share them with a friend that will hold you accountable. If you don't do this, it will be way too easy to cheat. You'll cut your fasts short and push them off for a tomorrow that never comes. You have to make a proclamation.

The Greek word *kērýssō* means to herald (proclaim); to preach (announce) a message publicly (Strong's Greek). This is the word used in Luke 4:18 (NIV) when Jesus tells the people in the synagogue that He came to "proclaim freedom for the prisoners." Your proclamation can't be a secret you keep to yourself or you won't stick to it. You don't have to shout it from the rooftops to impress anyone, but you do have to let at least one friend know so they'll hold you to your word.

I've seen people make decisions to fast without a firm commitment and break down as soon as someone invites them to a potluck. They don't have the resolve to bring a dish and not eat.

Step Three: Consider fasting with one or two close friends. This is something that will really help you stay committed, focused, and encouraged during your fast!

Step Four: Ask God to reveal to you the reasons He is calling you to fast and identify your specific areas of focus for the fast.

Step Five: Begin preparing your heart:

1. Fast to get God's attention

2. Kneel down in humility and ask for mercy and compassion

3. Pray continuously, "Lord, I believe. Help my unbelief!"

Then, make practical steps to prepare for your fast. Prepare your mind and your schedule. Fasting has physical challenges besides hunger. It can cause your breath to smell bad, you may get lightheaded, or it may make you even feel tired. I tend to go to bed by 8:00pm because my energy drops by then. Sometimes your brain is clearer, but sometimes it's foggier. Sometimes you may feel cranky or short-tempered. You could get a headache. Sensations will come and go in waves. Rip out the scripture cards in the back of this book to carry with you. When you feel any one of these things, say those scriptures to yourself. One of my favorites is:

Philippians 1:6 (NIV)

⁶ being confident of this, that he who began a good work in you will carry it on to completion until the day of Christ Jesus.

As a side note, while you don't want to be legalistic, you don't want to violate one rule in order to fulfill another one. I have seen people who will eat everything but the kitchen sink right before they fast. They gorge on everything they can because in their mind, they say "I am about to fast, so it's okay to overeat." But I believe the Bible says we should never overeat; we should put a knife to our throat if we are given to gluttony. Just like you can't break the law of stealing and justify it because you are going to do something good with the money, you can't overeat in order to prepare to fast.

Chapter 6
TYPES OF FASTS AND FASTING FOUND IN THE BIBLE

PART 1: TYPES OF FASTS

Before you begin your fast, you will need to commit to what type of fast you will be doing.

In the Bible, there are all kinds of different fasts. Some are 3 days, some are 40 days, some fasts are just for food, and some are for food and water. There are two types of Daniel fasts in the Bible, and we are going to talk about those later in this section. But for now, these are the main types of fasts that I will be referring to in this book. I broke them down into phases:

Phase 0) Dry Fast – This is no food. No water. The benefit of this is when you deprive your body of water, it has to pull water from other cells and go into survival of the fittest. All the weak cells die off and the powerful cells draw water from the weak cells. This is also really good for inflammation, even if it is short term. Fat has hydrogen in it, and hydrogen and oxygen make water. So if you are deprived of water, your body is going to create water from fat cells.

This is not the fast that we're practicing in this book. I call this fast Phase Zero because it is not something that I will recommend or talk about in this book. I just want you to know it exists.

Phase 1) Water Fast- You literally eat nothing but water

Phase 2) Coffee and Tea Fast- Only black coffee and unsweetened tea

Phase 3)The Limited Liquid Fast or Stabilizing Liquid Fast

With this fast I am drinking things that stabilize me, sustain me, and help take my fast to the next level:

- Water with one lemon or lime squeezed, or water with one freshly squeezed orange. This is only like .5 oz of freshly squeezed juice

- Organic Coffee with MCT Oil, Coconut Oil, Or a Non- Dairy Coconut Creamer like Laird Superfood

- Bone Broth- Bone broth is something that I use when I am doing longer fasts because it helps balance your electrolytes. Even though I am a fan of electrolyte packets, it seems like bone broth works even better.

Keep in mind that bone broth can be super high in sodium, so if you step on the scale when you are drinking a lot of bone broth, don't be surprised if you see your weight go up. I don't want you to weigh yourself during the fast and think you are destroying your metabolism.

- Organic Unsweetened Matcha Green Tea with Macadamia Nut Milk or Organic Canned Coconut Milk **Check the Can to make sure there is no Guar Gum or other chemicals like Carogean and sweeteners. It is really important that you are reading the labels on anything you add to your drinks during this phase. I was shocked when I was at Starbucks and asked to see the ingredients in their coconut milk. I couldn't believe all the chemicals and sweeteners. You want to keep your fast as clean as possible. If possible, make your own nut milks using only the nuts and water.

4. The Clean Juice and Smoothie Fast

I want to put a disclaimer that I do better when I am sticking to stabilizing drinks. These are drinks that help to stabilize your blood sugar. Even juices that are green, because they have fiber and proteins, will cause your blood sugar to spike and this will make you hungry. So, the benefit is that you are feeding your body nutrients and if you suffer with autoimmune issues like I do, these nutrients can help heal you on a longer fast. But be prepared that these juices and smoothies rev you up to a certain extent.

Throughout this book, I am going to refer to these different fasts and phases, so bookmark this page for easy reference!

When you are choosing your type of fast and length of fast, I want to encourage you to pray and seek God about how He would like you to fast, and what kind of fast he is calling you to do. Recently, the pastor at my church, Thomas Lane, announced that we were going to embark on a 21 day corporate fast during which everyone was supposed to give up something for 21 days. He said that everyone should pray and decide what they wanted to give up, maybe one meal, maybe social media. I knew that giving up one meal a day would not be a sacrifice for me, so I went for a really big sacrifice. Since I believe that the Biblical word for fasting means "to not eat," I decided that I was going to fast for 21 days by only drinking water, tea and coffee. The fast started out rough, and I expected to hit my stride, but when I got to day 7 of nothing but coffee, tea, and water, I noticed that my health was really declining. There's a difference between feeling uncomfortable and feeling ill, and I felt very ill. I felt like I was losing my mind and bodily functions. I prayed and asked God how He wanted me to move forward with my fast. I am not a quitter, and this was really hard for me to do. But I asked Him to give me clarity about how I should finish my fast and He gave me peace. I felt like He was telling me that I should transition from Phase 2, the water fast, with coffee and tea only, to the Phase 3 Fast to include stabilizing liquids. I want to be really clear that it is important to be in tune with the Holy Spirit and ask Him to guide your fast. Because I have so many health issues, I did not feel it was wise to continue past seven days; I literally felt like I could not function. It is important to keep your commitments, but sometimes you have to show yourself grace and evaluate and adjust. The biggest piece of this is to seek God's guidance if you feel He may be calling you to a long term fast. The reason He gave me peace about modifying my fast and including the stabilizing liquids is because even with these liquids added, 21 days is still a huge sacrifice and test of my faith. Stabilizing liquids do just enough to sustain you and allow you to function when you have reached your limits.

EATING AND FASTING IN THE BIBLE

I love Rick Warren, he is one of my favorite pastors to listen to and I have just learned so much from him. He created a fasting program called the Daniel Plan, which is very popular in Christian circles, and many churches do it together as a corporate fast. If you look this plan up, you'll see that it consists of 50% non starchy veggies, 25% lean proteins (animal or veggie proteins), 25% whole grains or starchy veggies, pasta, quinoa, beans, fruit. It allows things like healthy sweeteners, dark chocolate, etc.

The problem with the Daniel Plan is that it is a man-made diet. I know several people that gained weight doing this plan, because they were eating all this whole wheat pasta and beans. But more than that, they defeated the purpose of fasting which is taking the focus off food. Instead of focusing on their fast, they were focusing on finding all the foods they were allowed to eat and creating substitutes for the food they couldn't have. I went to the Bible to see what it has to say about the Daniel Plan. There are actually two types of fasts mentioned in Daniel.

I continued to study the book of Daniel and was blown away when I learned that they weren't talking about things like whole wheat pasta and meats in the Daniel plan. The first portion was strictly water and vegetables!

Let's read the full passage:

Daniel 1:11-17 (NIV)

[11] Daniel then said to the guard whom the chief official had appointed over Daniel, Hananiah, Mishael and Azariah, [12] "Please test your servants for ten days: Give us nothing but vegetables to eat and water to drink.[13] Then compare our appearance with that of the young men who eat the royal food, and treat your servants in accordance with what you see."[14] So he agreed to this and tested them for ten days.

[15] At the end of the ten days they looked healthier and better nourished than any of the

young men who ate the royal food. [16] So the guard

took away their choice food and the wine they were

to drink and gave them vegetables instead.

[17] To these four young men God gave knowledge

and understanding of all kinds of literature and

learning. And Daniel could understand visions and

dreams of all kinds.

First off, vegetables only, for ten days. Not even any fruit. The other observation here is the clarity that the men got, with knowledge and understanding, visions and dreams.

The second Daniel fast is in Chapter 10:2-3 (NIV)

[2] At that time I, Daniel, mourned for three weeks. [3]

I ate no choice food; no meat or wine touched my

lips; and I used no lotions at all until the three

weeks were over.

In my opinion, if you want to do a Daniel fast, I would do ten days of nothing but vegetables, then for three weeks after that, you would pray and consider what is choice food for you, and cut that out. For me, choice food would be things like sweets and snacks. For some it may be things like steak and cheese. Maybe cookies or brownies, wine or alcohol. I prayed about what I could get rid of. A slice of Ezekiel bread is something that I really, really love. That is definitely a choice food for me. Fruits veggies, and some nuts are all I need to sustain me and give me the nutrients I need. To me, there are no fruits or veggies you couldn't have except corn, which is a grain. As for liquids, you could have fresh pressed vegetable juice, coconut milk or almond milk. Preferably your nuts will be organic, raw and sprouted. Other foods to avoid would be sweeteners, breads, pasta, crackers, cookies, energy drinks, dairy products, candy, and meat. If you are going to use oil, you would use things like avocado oil, coconut oil, veggie oil, ghee, but definitely no corn oil.

So you should pray about what your choice foods are and cut those out. You need to eat only the substances God created for food, which he lists in Genesis 1:29 (NIV).

My regimen of what I did to really heal my body when I was very sick, was five days with just water and coffee, and then moved to ten days of vegetables, and three weeks of fruits, veggies, and nuts. After that, I added clean meats into my diet.

Leviticus 11:3 (NIV) You may eat any animal that has a divided hoof and that chews the cud.

Animals that chew the cud literally chew and swallow their food, then regurgitate a portion and chew it a second time. So, it's nice and clean.

Sheep, goat, deer, ox and cow are animals that chew the cud and have split hooves.

Other animals like horses and rabbits are unclean because they don't have split hooves.

Camel, rabbit, pig and squirrels are also unclean because they don't chew the cud.

An animal that is a scavenger eats everything they can find, even things that aren't suitable as food, so they have toxins, tape worms, parasites and viruses. Why would you want to eat that?

Leviticus 11:9 (NIV) "Of all the creatures living in the water of the seas and the streams you may eat any that have fins and scales."

You are to detest all of the things living in the water. That means shrimp, crab, and lobsters have toxins, harmful bacteria, parasites, and viruses. What happens is in our sewage systems we have so many chemicals, toxins, and bacteria, and those viruses and parasites get concentrated in the shellfish.

First of all, meat contains proteins, iron, Zinc, B6, B12 and Omega Fatty acids. I know a lot of people may be vegan or vegetarian. If God has led you to be vegan or vegetarian, by all means, just pray about it and if that's what you are allowed to do, then do that.

One of the things that is unfortunately in our food now is growth hormones, steroids, and antibiotics. The meat industry has been overfeeding and adding chemical stimulation to animals to get them bigger because they couldn't keep up with the meat demand.

As for myself, I eat meat but am particular about the quality. I make sure it's grass fed with no antibiotics, and I am not overdoing it.

Luke 24:42- (NKJV)- broiled fish and honeycomb

Proverbs 24:13 (NIV) Eat honey, my son, for it is good; honey from the comb is sweet to your taste.

There are 61 mentions of honey alone in the Bible!
Here are a couple verses of what God says to eat:

Genesis 1:29 (NIV)

Genesis 3:18 (NIV) [3] ... and you will eat the plants of the field

Ezekiel 16:19 (NIV) [19] Also the food I provided for you- the flour, olive oil and honey I gave you to eat- you offered as fragrant incense before them. That is what happened, declares he Sovereign Lord.

Genesis 43:11 (NIV) [11] Then their father Israel said to them, "If it must be, then do this: Put some of the best products of the land in your bags and take them down to the man as a gift—a little balm and a little honey, some spices and myrrh, some pistachio nuts and almonds.

Judges 7:13 (NIV)

Ezekial 4:9 (NIV) "Take wheat and barley, beans and lentils, millet and spelt; put them in a storage jar and use them to make bread for yourself

Proverbs 27:27 (NIV) You will have plenty of goats' milk to feed your family and to nourish your female servants.

Samuel 16:2 (NIV) [2] The king asked Ziba, "Why have you brought these?" Ziba answered, "The donkeys are for the king's household to ride on, the bread and fruit are for the men to eat, and the wine is to refresh those who become exhausted in the wilderness."

Leviticus 11:10 (NIV) "Of all the creatures living in the water of the seas and the streams you may eat any that have fins and scales."

Everyone is like you can have this, can't have that, don't eat this, don't eat that. I believe that when I read the Bible- fruits, veggies, nuts, meat that we mentioned, fish, milk, dairy are all acceptable for food. However, I believe that if the foods are altered and modified they lose a lot of their benefits and can cause sickness.

1 Corinthians 10:23 (NIV) "I have the right to do anything," you say—but not everything is beneficial. "I have the right to do anything"—but not everything is constructive.

I had to ask myself, even though I am permitted to eat these foods- how do I feel when I am eating them? How do I feel after I eat them?

As you know, I do a ton of podcasting, and a lot of the different guests that I have on my podcast encourage the listeners to ditch grains and take them out of the diet for the sake of their health. The two things that the health practitioners on our show (keep in mind they are usually naturopath, functional medicine doctors) say not to eat are grains and dairy. I've had different listeners and people in my Bible study that I host ask me over and over "If bread and grains are not good for you, why are they talked about so much in the Bible, and why does Jesus give so many references to bread and grains?" How could you say that bread is bad for you if Jesus is the bread of life? It was such a good point and personally, when I eat no grains at all, I am literally like a new person. It's like night and day how I feel when I eat grains and when I don't. I really had to battle this and say, "Okay, that is true. I can give you so many examples of the Bible mentioning barley and grains."

If grains are so unhealthy, why does the Bible refer to grains and bread and why does Jesus himself call himself the bread of life. It really is a huge point and I've researched this and read some different books on grains. After reading books and articles online about grains, here is the bottom line.

The way that they prepared grains in the Bible is completely different than the way they prepare grains today. In Bible times, grains were prepared by sprouting, fermenting and soaking them. If you think about the equipment that we have today to grind the grain to make flour, you will realize we don't have the same machines today as they had back then. Back then, grains were ground by hand or stones. The flour that we are eating today is ground at such a small size that your body then converts it to sugar. This is why flour in processed foods has such a big impact on our blood sugar. You've seen different studies in which a piece of bread could raise your blood sugar more than just eating straight sugar because of the way it's bleached and processed.

The grains in Biblical time wouldn't have been mixed with all these chemical additives! My husband jokes if you want Chantel to fall asleep in 10 minutes, give her a slice of bread. It will put me in bed the rest of the day! Know thy self … I know that for me, while other people can eat grains just fine, I can't.

The gist of all these different books and articles is that you should not eat grains and breads. After reading these books, the gist of the book is that the Bible was written during a very different agricultural time and the grains that were made thousands of years ago have little to no resemblance to the grains we are eating today. In Jesus' day, the grains had a higher protein content. If you looked and said "Okay here is a grain from Bible times and a grain from today", what would that look like? Not only are they totally different, but because they are trying to avoid pests, they are literally putting massive amounts of pesticides on all of this wheat. The wheat is sprayed with the same chemicals that are proven to kill rodents! How do you think our body is going to handle digesting that? It's no wonder why everyone has these autoimmune and gut issues! So, the grains in Jesus' time weren't even genetically similar to the grains we are eating today. And after having all of these chemicals sprayed upon them, why would you want to eat them?

The other piece that I want to note is that when I was looking at all the passages in the Bible about grains, it seemed like a lot of the verses that talked about grains were in the times of hardship. If someone was going through a hard time, they ate grains. It made me think of when I was in college; literally, I was so poor because I had no job and spent all the money my parents gave me on going to parties, so I had no money for groceries. The cheapest thing that we could eat was grilled cheese sandwiches. I can barely eat a grilled cheese sandwich to this day because of how many I had in college. A grilled cheese is extraordinarily cheap. You could buy a loaf of bread back then for $.89 and a pack of cheese on sale for $.99. So, for two dollars you could eat grilled cheese sandwiches for dinner for a week! Where it really talks about grains a lot is in the book of Ezekiel, and during the time this book was written, it was not a good time! There was a war and famine going on, and Ezekiel was told to eat carefully portioned amounts to be sure there was enough food. So in Ezekiel 4:1-17 (NIV) there's was an impending siege and the barley, lentil, and millet were the main things they had. His instructions were to weigh out the 20 shekels of food and eat it at set times during the 390 days. One of my favorite breads is Ezekiel bread, I don't eat grains often at all anymore because of how I feel. But if you are to eat bread, Ezekiel is one of the best! But if you read Ezekiel you're like WOW this is not a happy time!

In another story, God sent manna from heaven and they were eating manna every single day, and they were like "We can't eat manna anymore!" Then God gave them quail and meat.

Another example is during the seven years of famine in Egypt. When Joseph became prime minister, he only had seven years of plenty and stored up grains, so that is all they had to eat during the famine!

Basically, the bottom line is this, when there were bad times they ate whole grains because they had less meat and less fruits and veggies. When things were good, they ate meat, fruits and veggies. And actually, if you think about it in the Bible, meat is linked with celebration. When the prodigal son returned home to his father, what did he do instantly? He killed the fattened calf in celebration. He didn't suggest baking a loaf of bread! If you think about Passover, in the Old Testament meat sacrifices were often required, and I believe that in times of fasting, just like with Daniel taking out all meat and just eating veggies, there are massive benefits to fasting and removing proteins and fats for a certain amount of time. I know that Catholics, during Lent and other times, will sacrifice and give up something like meat. But meat in the Bible is tied up with celebration!

The final point of the whole Jesus is the bread of life argument, is that this is a metaphor explaining that he wants you to ingest him into your whole body and not just have head knowledge of him. You are eating the bread and consuming the bread, not just having head knowledge of it. Know what it tastes like! I could eat the most amazing chocolate chip cookie and describe it to my friend in great detail, but it wouldn't be the same as her tasting it for herself. It's the same with Jesus being the bread of life. I can describe Him to you, I can tell you what it's like to be in a personal relationship with Him and what it's like to experience Him, but you have to taste and see for yourself to really understand.

Chapter 7
PRACTICAL TIPS AND FASTING PLANS

For obvious reasons, Satan doesn't want you to fast! And he will do everything he can to stop you, even before you get started. In the time that I have attended my church, my pastor has never once missed a Sunday or "called out sick". One Sunday, he was going to introduce the church to the idea of a 21 day corporate fast, and he woke up with the stomach flu so bad that he had to miss his very first Sunday. God is hard at work at my church, and I believe this was just a small thwart of Satan to try to stop him. Since the devil is at work, we've got to work even harder to remain steadfast and strong before, during, and after our fast.

I want to share some of the really practical things that I've learned will help me while I fast. For example, you have to be really careful when you watch TV. Whenever I fast, without fail, I turn on the TV and the commercials are literally Papa John's pizza with buttery crusts and oozing cheese. This makes it extremely difficult to turn down and causes you to crave other foods that you are not eating. If you want to watch tv, watch something like Netflix or Hulu without commercials!

As I mentioned earlier, a lot of people gorge before they begin a fast. This means eating a lot in a short amount of time before you begin your fast. However, that is actually one of the worst things you can do! You should taper off your food intake right before a fast. Slowly adjust your intake going into the fast so that it is not as much of a complete shock to your body as if you stopped cold turkey. The whole point of a fast is to break the chains of addiction, so the last thing you want to do is be gluttonous right before a fast.

Remember that when you fast, you are going to get hungry! So many people tell me they can't fast because they feel too hungry. Yes, you will get hungry, and yes, it will be difficult, but I believe that it is truly one of the most amazing things you can do for yourself.

As soon as you decide to fast, things will spring up to get in the way. There will be dinners, parties, and more to throw you off track. Plan out your schedule. Don't schedule your fast to coincide with strenuous activities like personal training sessions or big social events like a wedding. You want to fast in a stress-free environment, both mentally and physically. If you know you're going to be slammed at work for a few days, don't plan a fast that same week. Avoid situations where people will be eating in front of you as much as you can.

This past Saturday, at the time of writing this book, was a perfect example of bad scheduling for me. I was on a fast but I had the bright idea to have my neighbors over for a cookout. I'm standing there making delicious grass-fed burgers and my favorite salad with cilantro and I was in torture the entire time. You don't have to do that to yourself. Plan ahead.

Another time when I was fasting, I was scheduled to have dinner at my favorite restaurant, Le Yaca, with one of my managers, Heather Roemmich, as a prize for a work contest. The only problem was in the middle of a three day fast! This fast had been super easy for me, but here at the last leg came this roadblock. When I realized that I messed up my schedule, I asked God to find a way to cancel it or let me end the fast early. I did not want to have to go to Le Yaca and watch Heather eat my favorite steak in front of me!

Later, Heather texted me that she was exhausted from a vacation she just got back from and wanted to spend time with her husband. She postponed! It was an answered prayer.

Make the commitment and try to push through. Not eating something you want isn't the end of the world. The restaurant will still be there and you will eat again.

I ran into another challenge tonight when my husband asked me to cook him eggs and biscuits. Sidenote: I make the best eggs in town. The secret is low and slow. Egg and cheese biscuits are one of the hardest things for me to resist. My husband offered to make them himself because he knew I was fasting, but I wanted to do it for him anyway. Big mistake! I resisted but I shouldn't have put myself through the temptation.

Don't put yourself in tempting situations when you fast. Sometimes you'll feel weak and other times you'll feel strong and motivated. When you're weak, don't make your favorite food!

I can't stress enough how difficult it is to fast. It's not something you can do using your own strength, so you have to rely on strength from God to make it through.

It still amazes me that it was food that enticed Adam and Eve to sin. The fall of mankind was all because of a piece of fruit! On the flip side, Jesus began his whole ministry with a fast. It amazes me that when I tell Christians I'm fasting they tell me they could never do it themselves. Christians downplay the importance of fasting even though it opens the door to a more powerful and intimate relationship with God. It's not until you do it that you understand how close it brings you to Him. After just a couple of days of fasting you feel that power that you can only get from Him. If Jesus felt the need to fast to begin His ministry, how much more do we need to fast?

I am beginning a ministry with the Lord reaching out to people and helping them with their eating. That's part of the reason I'm fasting more.

Hebrews 4:15 (NIV)

15 For we do not have a high priest who is unable to empathize with our weaknesses, but we have one who has been tempted in every way, just as we are—yet he did not sin.

Because Jesus fasted, He can sympathize with how hard it truly is to fast.

Hebrews 4:16 (NIV)

16 Let us then approach God's throne of grace with confidence, so that we may receive mercy and find grace to help us in our time of need."

With these promises, we know we can succeed. This is such a powerful verse for you to say when you're on a fast.

Now, once you decide that fasting is something you need to do, don't try to substitute fasting food with fasting something else. A lot of people fast Facebook, TV, or video games, but it is not the same. Fasting food is what takes you to the next level. Fasting other things is great but remember that the Greek word for "fast" means "not to eat." This is the fasting the Bible talks about.

Think about the fact that one third of the world goes to bed hungry. If you're a Christian who doesn't believe in fasting, I would argue big time that you need to look at the Scripture again because that is an incorrect viewpoint.

Fasting is not abstaining from food because food is sinful in and of itself. In the Bible, people fasted by abstaining from food, and when it was over, they went right back to eating. As I am writing this, it's Easter and a lot of people are giving up things for a season for Lent. I've heard people say they are giving up all kinds of things for Lent. They say they are giving up gossip, lying, holding grudges, being unkind, all kinds of stuff. All of these things they are giving up for Lent are actual sins. In the Bible, when you fast, you go back to eating when the fast is over. So while giving up all of these things is great, they don't constitute a fast. The idea with sin is that you kill it daily, you die to it daily.

Matthew 6:2, 5, 16 (NIV)

² "So when you give to the needy, do not announce it with trumpets, as the hypocrites do in the synagogues and on the streets, to be honored by

others. Truly I tell you, they have received their reward in full.

5 "And when you pray, do not be like the hypocrites, for they love to pray standing in the synagogues and on the street corners to be seen by others. Truly I tell you, they have received their reward in full.

16 "When you fast, do not look somber as the hypocrites do, for they disfigure their faces to show others they are fasting. Truly I tell you, they have received their reward in full.

Do you see those three scriptures? Jesus gave fasting just as much priority as he did giving and praying. If you have time to do the other two, then you have time to fast.

I feel more passionate now about fasting than I ever have in my entire life. Don't get me wrong, there is nobody that loves food more than me! I love to eat and I'm a true foodie. I have to constantly remind myself that hungering for God is so much better than food. Yes, that steak from Le Yaca is amazing, but it's so much better to eat food from the Lord and draw on His strength and power.

Matthew 5:6 (NIV)

6 Blessed are those who hunger and thirst for righteousness, for they will be filled.

Because I'm so hungry right now, I've been repeating this scripture over and over again. When you develop a hunger for the deeper things and a more intimate relationship with God, He fills you up. Sometimes, doing the regular, monotonous things over and over again just doesn't do it.

TRANSITIONING INTO YOUR FAST AND SAMPLE FASTING PLANS

I mentioned previously in this chapter that I dived straight in to my first extended fast head first, and it was a disaster!

To help you understand how you can build up to a long fast, I created a sample 3 month outline.

Week 1: Start with a 6 hour eating window for 5 days (Fasting 18 hours per day)

Week 2: Complete one 24 hour fast (I recommend fasting from dinner to dinner, or lunch to lunch, so you could start your fast after dinner on Wednesday and eat again at dinner on Thursday. Or, start your fast after lunch on Friday and eat again at lunch on Saturday.)

Week 3: One 48 hour fast

Week 4: 3 Day Fast

Week 5: 6 Hour eating window for 5 days

Week 6: One 24 hour fast

Week 7: One 48 hour fast

Week 8: 5 day fast

Week 9: 6 hour eating window for 5 days

Week 10: One 24 hour fast

Week 11: One 48 hour fast

Week 12: 7 day fast

Feel free to try this in its entirety, to shorten it, or extend it! Pray and ask God how long he is calling you to fast.

TRANSITIONING OUT OF YOUR FAST

The longer your fast, the more important your transition **out** of your fast is. If I just finished a three day fast, the last thing I want to do is eat a big steak and mashed potatoes as my first meal.

Your transition should be half the time of your fast.

3 Day Fast: 1 ½ Day Transition

4 Day Fast: 2 Day Transition

6 Day Fast: 3 Day Transition

8 Day Fast: 4 Day Transition

Be careful with processed ingredients and animal products during your transition. You just finished cleansing your body of a lot of toxins, so be careful of what you put back in. Fats and animals are harder to digest. I even eat fruits and vegetables separately and pair proteins with non-starchy vegetables. Different combinations digest better than others. I don't want you to stress about food combining, but some things are common sense. Have a big ol' burger and fries and you'll feel terrible. The very first thing I try to eat after I break a long fast is a smoothie that is mostly vegetables. Then I might have some fruits or cooked vegetables. I, personally, stick to pretty much fruits and vegetables after a long fast.

Recently I was coming off a long fast and on the first day I was away on a business trip and I wanted to eat at two of my favorite restaurants, True Food Kitchen and the Nordstrom Café. One restaurant for lunch, and one for dinner, and both times I ordered my absolute favorite dishes, both of which had meat on them! Both dishes sounded amazing but as soon as they got to the table, I couldn't stand the smell or taste of the meat. I just couldn't eat it, and I am not sure why! I just listened to my body and stuck to the veggies. Listen to what your body is telling you that you can handle!

FASTING DIGESTION AND SIDE EFFECTS

It's possible to experience bad breath as a result of fasting. This happens for a few possible reasons. One, your body produces less saliva when you're not eating. That saliva helps break down bacteria in your mouth. There's less saliva available to do that when you're fasting. The smell can also come from bacteria in your digestive fluids in your stomach. There are also toxins leaving your body while you fast that can contribute to the problem. Keep mouthwash handy and floss more than you normally would.

You may also develop a white film on your tongue. Use a tongue scraper or a toothbrush to clean that off. Another big side effect is headaches if you're not having any caffeine on your fast. Sometimes, people forget to drink water and they get dehydrated. You could feel symptoms of low blood sugar because you're not consuming sugar and your glucose is down.

Another side effect is extreme emotions. Fasting doesn't just rid your body of toxins; it can bring up repressed emotions you've been stuffing down. You can no longer hide behind the food and those emotions rise to the surface. You may feel more emotional, "hangry," sad, or want to cry. All of these are natural and the best thing to do is pray about it, go for a long walk, or take a bath instead of running to food.

Eating food is a process of digestion, assimilation, and elimination of waste. You have four organs of elimination: your bowels, kidneys, lungs, and skin. No matter how light or healthy the food you eat is, it takes work for it to pass through your gastrointestinal tract and be eliminated from your body. That's why a water fast is so necessary. You have to give your body a break so it can have internal purification.

Even if you're a healthy eater, your food can be covered in poisons from pesticides and toxic fertilizers. If you want proof of what I'm talking about, you can fill up a cup with a sample of your own urine and let it sit for a while. You'll see crystals form in it. If you were to have the sample studied, they would find traces of pesticides in your urine. Fasting removes these poisons from your body. Knowing that will excite you and keep you going while you fast. You're healing your body from the inside out.

MELTDOWN MODE

When I am fasting most of the time, I have all this energy and clarity and I am like "This is the best day ever!" And there are other times that my staff calls "Meltdown Mode." They can see it in my eyes, I start staring in space, I am so tired, and I have no energy! My staff starts laughing at me because sometimes I can't complete my thoughts or things I say don't make sense. They will ask if I need a coconut water from Whole Foods or what they can do to help!

When you are extremely tired during a fast, there are several reasons:

1) Electrolyte and mineral deficiency

You need to have balanced electrolytes. When your kidneys detect that you have less insulin in your body, it flushes water out. You can tell when you fast that you pee a lot because it flushes you out. If you drink too much water, your electrolytes will be unbalanced. So the first thing I will do, if I am being extraordinarily strict, is put some salt in my water if I am sodium deficient. I will also take these Nuun hydration capsules. They do have 15 calories and some of them have around 2g of sugar, but they have a ton of minerals and electrolytes.

Your kidneys excrete minerals from your body to be sure you have the right balance, so you want to be sure you have the right potassium. Whenever I have my meltdowns, I know my potassium is low. When I take potassium and iron, I feel like a new person. Another tip is right before I start my fast, I like to eat foods that are high in potassium like avocados and potatoes.

The seven major electrolytes in your body are sodium, chloride, potassium, magnesium, calcium, phosphate, and bicarbonate. The three most important being sodium, magnesium, and potassium. So, taking an electrolyte tablet when you are fasting is important because when I get in complete and utter meltdown mode and take an electrolyte tablet, it really helps me.

2)Lack of Movement

When you are tired and don't feel good, you just want to lay down! But that is not going to make you feel better. What will make you feel better is to go for a walk! Especially in the middle of the day when I am in meltdown mode, getting Vitamin D and going for a walk is the best thing for me. Have you ever gone to the gym tired, and when you leave, you actually have more energy? Crazy how it works!

3) Fuel Transition

When you start fasting, it takes your body a while to go from burning sugar to fat. Your body has to adapt to burning fat instead of glycogen for fuel! You want your body to be using its reserved fat for fuel. When your body is in the transition from one fuel source to the other, you get really tired. Once you tap out of your sugar reserves and start using your fat for fuel, that's when you have more energy and clarity and are more alert. It's the transition time that can be rough. For me, I know that Day 2 and Day 3 of my fast are very difficult because if you think about it, your body has hundreds of thousands of calories of fat just sitting there in your body. Say you give your body 2,000 calories per day. The best analogy I can think of is from a show I saw last night in which they were serving beer kegs, and when one keg was emptied or tapped out, they had to switch to a new keg and serve that. So when your sugar keg taps out, your body moves to your fat keg, but it takes a little time to switch out the kegs and transition.

Chapter 8
NO EXCUSES

You can always find a reason not to fast:

"I have a party"

"I forgot about his lunch meeting."

"It's my anniversary."

I recently went on a walk with my friend Stephanie and was talking to her about fasting. She said, "I want to do some more fasting, the main reason is to lose weight". One of the things that she was worried about was her schedule. The next day, she had small group and there are always snacks. And she knew people would ask why she wasn't eating them, and she would have to tell them she was fasting. The next day she had a dinner planned with someone, the following day a lunch with someone. I told her that yesterday I went out to lunch with three friends, and we went to Aldos, one of my favorite restaurants in Virginia Beach. I didn't eat anything but hot water with lemon. Later that night, I sat with my family while they ate dinner. I've gone to literally hundreds of lunches and dinners where I didn't eat, either because I wasn't physically hungry or because I was fasting. The main thing you have to do is change your mindset! I went in with the mindset that I am not eating, and it's not that big of a deal. I am going to use this time to spend time talking to my friends. I am still having fun, still enjoying myself! Instead of shoving food in my face I get to connect and bond with people I enjoy being with. Every once in a while I will go to another place that my girlfriends love in Virginia Beach called Stock Pot. If I am fasting, I will get a bowl of their chicken noodle soup with no chicken and no noodles, and just enjoy the broth.

There's a Benjamin Franklin quote I love that says "He that is good at making excuses is seldom good for anything else". The bottom line is you could literally make an excuse to get out of fasting anytime. If you're a busy person and you have a lot of friends, you will have a different excuse every single week on why you aren't going to fast, just like my friend Stephanie. She looked at me like a deer in headlights when I told her that I go to restaurants and don't eat!

Recently I went to New York City to meet a CEO of another real estate company who took me to dinner at Nobu. My husband took me there in Miami and without alcohol, the meal was like $400! This place is so nice, so delicious, and so expensive, it's like celebrity central! This would be a perfect example of a time where I could say, "I am going to break my fast just this once since someone is taking me to a really nice dinner at Nobu." But you can make excuses, or you can make it happen. There were about six people at dinner and they were ordering tons of food and passing it around, family style. After every dish that was passed around, everyone agreed that it was the best thing they had ever tasted. I was on the 9th day of an extended fast and was only drinking stabilizing liquids. I ordered some bone broth, and it was the nastiest bone broth I've ever tasted, so I didn't really drink it. I ended up just having hot water with lemon. I really focused on the conversation and had a great time! And, it was the craziest thing, even though the food looked great, God took away my desire to eat it and it didn't even smell good to me. At the time, I was fasting to ask the Lord to heal my body from my autoimmune issues and thyroid issues. I was also really fasting to take my business to the next level, to bring on high level leaders and scale our call center to go nationwide. These things are huge and really important for me. Much more important to me than a dinner at Nobu. I made the decision that the breakthroughs I would get from fasting outweighed a nice dinner out.

Luke 14:16-24 (NIV)

16 Jesus replied: "A certain man was preparing a great banquet and invited many guests. 17 At the time of the banquet he sent his servant to tell those who had been invited, 'Come, for everything is now ready.'

18 "But they all alike began to make excuses. The first said, 'I have just bought a field, and I must go and see it. Please excuse me.'

19 "Another said, 'I have just bought five yoke of oxen, and I'm on my way to try them out. Please excuse me.'

²⁰ "Still another said, 'I just got married, so I can't come.'

²¹ "The servant came back and reported this to his master. Then the owner of the house became angry and ordered his servant, 'Go out quickly into the streets and alleys of the town and bring in the poor, the crippled, the blind and the lame.'

²² "'Sir,' the servant said, 'what you ordered has been done, but there is still room.'

²³ "Then the master told his servant, 'Go out to the roads and country lanes and compel them to come in, so that my house will be full. ²⁴ I tell you, not one of those who were invited will get a taste of my banquet.'"

The people who didn't want to attend the banquet all made excuses. People make the same kind of excuses for why they can't fast.

Too old. Too young. Diabetic, etc. etc.

Luke 2:36-38 (NIV)

³⁶ There was also a prophet, Anna, the daughter of Penuel, of the tribe of Asher. She was very old; she had lived with her husband seven years after her marriage, ³⁷ and then was a widow until she was

eighty-four. She never left the temple but worshiped night and day, fasting and praying. [38] Coming up to them at that very moment, she gave thanks to God and spoke about the child to all who were looking forward to the redemption of Jerusalem.

Anna was an elderly person who fasted REGULARLY. Her fasting and prayer gave her a sensitivity to God that allowed her to perceive who Jesus was when everyone else missed why this Child was special. You're not too old to fast. In fact, I believe our elders should set the example for young people on prayer and fasting.

I've heard men in particular make the excuse that they work too hard to fast. I don't think that's true. I work out with heavy weight while fasting regularly and I know men who lift heavier weights than me with more active lifestyles and they fast too.

I know a lot of wives and mothers who tell me that they can't fast because they cook for their families and it's too hard to resist eating. I think that's a good time to send your family out to eat. Seriously, you can still cook and fast. It takes more strength, but you can do it. I do it often. I do it so much that when I did sit down to eat with my family one night, my son said, "Mom, you're eating with us? That's so great!" Pretty funny.

You need to write down all of your excuses and examine them. If it's a medical problem, realize that God is able to heal you. It's not like you have to go to the extreme right away. Talk to your doctor about it. You can start slow and work your way into it. If you're someone who takes medicine that has to be taken with food, then have something like a cracker.

Be like Nike. Stop making excuses. Just do it.

One of my favorite preachers is Carl Lentz, who has a really great ministry in New York City. Typically, I agree with everything he says, but recently, he went on The View, and made a statement that he got a lot of bad feedback on. The ladies on The View asked him if he thought abortion was sinful and he responded that people have to live with their own convictions and that he did not classify the issue as an "open and shut case". He later clarified after the interview and came out and said that he did believe abortion was a sin, but I was really disappointed, like many other Christians, that he did not take the opportunity to make a stand for the truth.

There are so many people out there who are saying that you need to live by your own convictions, just like this pastor. People say: "You do you, boo" or "You live your truth." But what if your truth is actually a lie? We have to align our truth with God's truth and what He says to us in His word.

On day 13 of a 14 day fast, I was feeling hungry. The final leg can be really hard. I decided to read the story of Jesus fasting in all three different gospels and see if I could learn anything different and new. This story is told three times, in the books of Matthew, Mark, and Luke. One of the things that I noticed is that Jesus was fasting before he went to the cross. Often times, Jesus will call you to fast in preparation for a trial that is right around the corner. I never noticed this about the scripture before.

Matthew 4:2 (NIV) made me laugh: "After fasting forty days and forty nights, he was hungry". I want to go ahead and nominate this as the most obvious verse in the Bible. If you don't eat for forty days, of course you will be hungry!

Another thing I noticed when I was re-reading the story of Jesus being tempted is that Jesus was tempted three times while He was fasting, and I noticed that this happens to me! I feel like my temptation comes in threes when I am fasting. Jesus responded to temptation by quoting three verses and I believe that we should do the same thing, memorize scriptures to combat this temptation.

But the biggest thing that stood out to me as I kept reading Matthew 4:1-25 (NIV) is that we always think that the devil only comes to us and tempts us with lies. But He's smarter than that. He knows that if we love God, we might recognize a lie really easily, and refuse to fall for it. So what he does sometimes is tempt you with the truth. In this passage of Matthew 4:1-25 (NIV), Jesus is hungry. He had been fasting for 40 days and what does the devil do? The devil goes in and what he did was attack with the Bible. He attacked him with the truth! He quoted scripture to Him and twisted that to use it against Him. We have to outsmart Satan and learn to recognize these truths.

It's crazy because a few days prior I was really struggling with hunger, so I decided to open the Bible and what did I read?

Ecclesiastes 9:7 (NIV) Go, eat your food with gladness, and drink your wine with a joyful heart, for God has already approved what you do.

Was God telling me to eat? No, He called me to fast. But Satan was trying to tempt me with these truths out of context.

Another one was Genesis 1:29 (NIV)

Then God Said, "I give you every seed-bearing plant on the face of the whole earth and every tree that has fruit with seed in it. They will be yours for food."

Genesis 9:3 (NIV) Everything that lives and moves about will be food for you. Just as I gave you the green plants, I now give you everything.

Here I was on this extended fast, and I knew that He called me to it, so a way the devil could tempt me was by saying "You need to eat food, your body needs the nutrients." Yes, this is true. Food does contain nutrients and we do need to fuel our bodies. That's not a lie! Did God create all these plants and fruits for me to eat? Yes. These are not lies. But, I knew that God called me to this fast, and that He and His truth would sustain me. I wasn't going to allow Satan to twist these verses to justify the temptation to break the fast that God called me to.

If you are grounded in God's truth, the Devil may be successful in getting you to commit a "big" sin, like cheating on your husband or stealing from your company, so he will begin to do whatever he can to get you to believe a little lie, sprinkled with a little truth and to get a stronghold by messing with your mindset.

I have a really great, Godly friend that I really admire. She is grounded in the word, and Satan has been unsuccessful in getting her to commit these "big sins," so he tries to tempt her with little truths and lies to make her less effective for the kingdom. One area that she really struggles with is making excuses. The other day she was telling me that she wanted to get her real estate license, but the problem is that she has been saying this for a really long time! I have people at my company who get their license in as little as two weeks, so I know that it can be done. She feels like she is called to become a real estate agent and the devil is planting little lies of excuses in her mind as to why she is too busy to do it, and it's always something! I am a "tell it like it is" friend, in case you can't tell, so when she was talking about this with me the other day, I told her she needed to stop making excuses and be like Nike "Just Do It". She's overwhelmed at the idea of getting her license, and I get that. So, I told her that what she needs to do is create a plan of attack! Set a timeline for herself, create accountability by finding people to hold her to that timeline, and create really specific action steps for how she's going to get there.

Satan wants her to live a defeated life, but I refuse to let a friend of mine fall for these excuses that are keeping her from what God has in store. I told her that for the next 30 days she has to really focus on her goals and getting her self- esteem back up by saying "I am going to win, no matter what, and anytime Satan throws an excuse in my face, I will respond "Not today, Satan!"

My friend was setting her goals too high, and really needed to break them down into tiny bites to build her confidence up by achieving her goals. I love tennis and I knew a girl that was playing with people just a little above her skill level. She was playing at a level 4 and was losing every single match, and felt so defeated. So she moved herself down to a 3.5 just for a little while, so she could remember what winning feels like! She needed to build up her confidence by winning again, and say "I am going to win, no matter what!"

Maybe for you, starting a 21 day fast sounds like a huge, impossible goal. Start with shorter, 24 hour fasts to build up your confidence and celebrate some wins!

The only way to outsmart the devil is by asking God to reveal the lies and the truths that he is tempting you with for what they are. Say it with me, "I am going to win, no matter what! No more excuses!"

PART 3

During Your Fast

Chapter 9
YOUR FAITH AND FASTING

You can get into a rut even if you pray and go to church every week. You can lack the power of God in your life and wonder why you're not seeing deliverance. One of the easiest meals for me to cook is spaghetti, so I cook it all the time. Because of this, my family is starting to get tired of it. Sometimes the same thing happens in our spiritual lives. We attend the same old church services and pray the same old prayers that we don't put much thought into. It becomes very mundane, like spaghetti. Fasting breaks you out of your monotony. Fasting is what I call a real faith builder.

When I fast, even the church service comes alive. I hear things more clearly and worship is more powerful. When I read the Bible, I'm like, "Whoa, I never saw that before!" One of my favorite verses is Romans 12:1.

Romans 12:1 (NIV)
12 Therefore, I urge you, brothers and sisters, in view of God's mercy, to offer your bodies as a living sacrifice, holy and pleasing to God—this is your true and proper worship.

Paul prayed three times in 2 Corinthians for God take away the thorn in his flesh. Three times isn't much compared to how many times I've prayed for that kind of thing!

2 Corinthians 12:9 (NIV)

⁹ But he said to me, "My grace is sufficient for you, for my power is made perfect in weakness." Therefore I will boast all the more gladly about my weaknesses, so that Christ's power may rest on me.

God's grace is all you need.

James 5:17-18 (NIV)

¹⁷ Elijah was a human being, even as we are. He prayed earnestly that it would not rain, and it did not rain on the land for three and a half years. ¹⁸ Again he prayed, and the heavens gave rain, and the earth produced its crops.

Sometimes, we think the heroes of the Bible are superhuman or somehow just not the same as us. But this passage says otherwise. Elijah was just like us. So, why did God give him more favor? I believe it's because he fasted and prayed. He controlled his appetite and made his assignment before God more important. The power of fasting and prayer unlocked a whole new level for him.

Every time I read the Bible now, I see something about fasting! The book of Luke talks about fasting as a way to enhance our walk with God and witness.

One of my favorite verses in the Bible is Joel 2:25-26 (NIV)

Joel 2:25-26 (NIV)

25 "I will repay you for the years the locusts have eaten—

the great locust and the young locust,

the other locusts and the locust swarm—

my great army that I sent among you.

26 You will have plenty to eat, until you are full,

and you will praise the name of the Lord your God,

who has worked wonders for you;

never again will my people be shamed.

This verse says to me that there are things that are not fair that come along in your life, but that God will restore your years and can turn things around. A perfect example is my husband. He had a very bad childhood. His dad was a drug addict and in jail. His mother was addicted to drugs and died of an overdose. None of that was fair for him, but I believe that he is the person he is today because of what he went through. It turned out to be a blessing. It's like with Joseph in the Bible. He went from being a slave to Prime Minister of Egypt. He would never have gotten there if his brothers hadn't sold him into slavery. Sometimes, God will put you into "jail" so He can take you to your purpose.

Genesis 50:20 (NIV)

20 You intended to harm me, but God intended it for good to accomplish what is now being done, the saving of many lives.

After God delivered the children of Israel out of Egypt, they were constantly tempted to turn around and go back. Why would they do this? Why would they willingly go back into slavery?

Numbers 11:5 (NIV)

5 We remember the fish we ate in Egypt at no cost—also the cucumbers, melons, leeks, onions and garlic.

It was food! All they could think about was their stomachs. God has called us to not be ruled by our appetites. If you want to live an abundant Christian life, you must not be a slave to your stomach.

SECRET FASTING

There are certain things that people expect Christians to be, and one is loving. We always say that we are brothers and sisters in Christ, and that we love people because we are children of God. Some other things that people assume Christians will do is give to the needy and pray. Those are kind of givens.

Even in the sermon on the Mount in Matthew 6:3 (NIV), it says "When you give to the needy," it is an assumption that Christians will be giving. It also says, "When you pray" and "When you fast." Again, it is assumed that these will be natural habits when you give your life to Christ.

It's funny that it never says, "When you read scripture" or "When you attend bible study," or "when you are meeting with other Christians," or even "when you are doing evangelism."

When I started to really study fasting, I was so shocked by the number of Christians who have never fasted a day in their life. Fasting is so different than any other acts like giving and prayer, because it's in a whole new realm of obedience. It is different because it's up to the believer to pray and ask God how long, how often and to what extent. There are no clear cut guidelines in the Bible on how long we should fast or how often.

In 1 Thessalonians 5: 16-18 (NIV), the Bible says, "Pray without ceasing," so that is super clear. We should live in a constant mindset and attitude of prayer and communication with God. But there's only one time in the Bible where God commanded a specific corporate fast on a specific day of the year.

Leviticus 23:27 (NIV) "The tenth day of this seventh month is the Day of Atonement. Hold a sacred assembly and deny yourselves,[a] and present a food offering to the LORD.

The one time a year God commanded the children of Israel to fast is in this verse of Leviticus. Basically, what this verse is saying is that this is a time to deny yourself again of food. Not Facebook, not Starbucks, not Netflix.

Even though the Bible doesn't lay out many specifics on how often or how long we should fast, it is very clear about something we shouldn't do while we are fasting.

Matthew 6:16 (NIV) When you fast, do not look somber as the hypocrites do, for they disfigure their faces to show others they are fasting. Truly I tell you, they have received their reward in full. [17] But when you fast, put oil on your head and wash your face, [18] so that it will not be obvious to others that you are fasting, but only to your Father, who is unseen; and your Father, who sees what is done in secret, will reward you.

One misconception about this verse is that it is saying that you shouldn't tell anyone about the fast. When I first read this passage, I thought it was saying that we should go out of our way to be sure no one finds out that we are fasting. If they do find out, my fast would be worthless. But we already know that according to the Old Testament, everyone should be fasting on Yom Kippur, so that wasn't a secret. Everyone knew that everyone else was fasting! Even as modern day Christians, we often do corporate fasts as a church. So we all know that our friends at church are fasting with us. In the Old Testament, Esther 4:16 (NIV) says "Go assemble all the Jews, do not eat or drink, me and my maidens will also fast."

Again, she is telling everyone that they are going to fast together as a group. In the New Testament, in Acts 14, the church fasted together before they sent Pau and Barnabas out. As a church, they fasted, prayed, laid hands on them, and sent them on their way. If someone finds out you are fasting, it's not a sin. The value of your fast is not destroyed because somebody knows. And there is definitely value in fasting with other believers!

Now, what does this passage actually mean? It means that being seen fasting and fasting to be seen are two different things. Fasting to be seen means you are going out of your way to say "Hey, look at me, I am fasting." You are going out of your way to make sure everyone knows that you are fasting. When you walk in the room, maybe you are even disfiguring your face to look weak and miserable so people ask you what's wrong. Unfortunately, I am one of those people that wears my heart on my sleeve and everyone sees it on my face when I am not feeling well, but I am not intentionally going around saying "Oh I am dying, poor me!"

The passage also says "Anoint your head and wash your face." So basically even while you are fasting, you get up and do your hair and makeup and look nice, you are making sure that you are taking care of yourself as you usually would. If you run around all the time looking pathetic, no one will ever want to fast! They will be think to themselves, "Oh my goodness, look what fasting does to a person. She looks like death; I don't want to do that!" Self- denial is a godly practice and you are denying yourself with the intention of getting closer to God. So while you are denying yourself, you should have extra joy and gladness and be filled with the Holy Spirit.

Recently, one of my friends asked another "Is Chantel eating today?" and the other replied that I was fasting, and she said "I am going to wait to talk to her until she's eating again". This was convicting for me when I heard this because an actual problem! When I am fasting, I should be filled with the Holy Spirit more than normal. I am spending more time in the word and more time with Him, so should be bubbling over with the Holy Spirit, not being a bear to my friends.

Don't get it twisted, there are going to be times in life that you are going to be sad and mourning. In Matthew 5:4 (NIV), the Bible says:

4 Blessed are those who mourn, for they will be comforted

You will be sad at times, but we aren't supposed to be purposefully to get attention, and you definitely don't want to cause a brother to stumble by seeing you so miserable that they never want to fast.

Chapter 10
Waiting for a Breakthrough

Matthew 7:7 (NIV)

7 "Ask and it will be given to you; seek and you will

find; knock and the door will be opened to you.

"I've been praying and fasting but still haven't gotten

a breakthrough."

I felt like this millions of times in my journey to lose weight. It was such a

struggle for so many years that I felt like I identified with the apostle Paul and

the "thorn" in his side.

2 Corinthians 12:6-10 (NIV)

6 Even if I should choose to boast, I would not be

a fool, because I would be speaking the truth. But

I refrain, so no one will think more of me than is

warranted by what I do or say, 7 or because of these

surpassingly great revelations. Therefore, in order

to keep me from becoming conceited, I was given a

thorn in my flesh, a messenger of Satan, to torment me. ⁸ Three times I pleaded with the Lord to take it away from me. ⁹ But he said to me, "My grace is sufficient for you, for my power is made perfect in weakness." Therefore I will boast all the more gladly about my weaknesses, so that Christ's power may rest on me. ¹⁰ That is why, for Christ's sake, I delight in weaknesses, in insults, in hardships, in persecutions, in difficulties. For when I am weak, then I am strong.

I thought maybe I was like Paul. If I had been skinny, maybe I would have become conceited. I thought that could be the reason why I couldn't lose weight. However, once I learned that overeating was a sin, I realized that wasn't true. This was something I had to overcome. Instead of making excuses for my problems, I needed to learn to be consistent.

In C.S. Lewis' *The Problem of Pain*, he said, "Pain insists upon being attended to. God whispers to us in our pleasures, speaks in our conscience, but shouts in our pain: it is His megaphone to rouse a deaf world."

God uses pain to get our attention and lead us into a breakthrough. If you're happy and content where you are, then there's no need for change. I have a friend who is over 300lbs but doesn't have a desire to lose weight. Why? Because he's in good health! He doesn't see the need to change. He enjoys eating as a hobby and he's overwhelmed at the idea of changing his routine. Without the pressure of pain, it's hard to change. Sometimes it takes a painful experience to force you to change your ways. When the pain in your life exceeds the fear of change, that's when you make a decision.

In what area of life do you need a breakthrough? Is it in your health? Finances? A relationship? Your emotional or mental state? Your job? Your relationship with God? Whatever the area of stagnation, you have to put your focus and energy into changing to see a breakthrough. You can't move into a breakthrough without moving first!

Psalm 77:2 (NIV)

² When I was in distress, I sought the Lord; at night
I stretched out untiring hands …

I love this passage! Imagine that visual of reaching out to God when you need Him more than anything. It's why fasting is so important. You're telling Him that you're serious about wanting a breakthrough.

Something that I have found is really crucial in this breakthrough is putting a stop to the blame game. I see this a lot when people are wounded and feeling inadequate, disregarded, unworthy, or not feeling good about themselves. They either retreat, attack, or freeze. When they are defensive, will often they will attack. But, when an animal is hurt, they hurt other animals! But other times, they will go in the corner and pee. So the person who is wounded emotionally, instead of physically, they will attack. But you have to be sensitive with them because they may feel inadequate or powerless, like things are out of their control. When things are out of their control, that's when they try to take the power back.

This is really common with married couples; someone says something and the other takes it the wrong way and will say something nasty in return.

Let's say a husband wants to sleep with his wife, and she doesn't want to sleep with him and she rejects him. What he is really feeling is unloved and rejection, but instead of saying "I feel rejected," he will probably attack and say, "You are a terrible wife. You never do anything for me. You are this and you are that." He will attack instead of saying, "this is how I felt, I felt unloved or rejected." And in return, she will attack him probably! It's a vicious cycle. If you are struggling with this vicious cycle, take a deep look within, and stop the blame game.

WHEN THE ANSWER IS NO

Fasting is not something you do to manipulate God. If you fast for something and you don't end up getting what you wanted, you can't get discouraged. Fasting doesn't manipulate God to do something that's not His will. It gets you ready for God's answer. It prepares you to do "not my will, but Yours." (Luke 22:42 NIV)

Fasting breaks you down to a position of total obedience and humility where you relinquish your life to Him and trust that He has your best interests at heart even when you don't understand.

There's a story of David in the Bible who fasted to save his son's life, and his son still died.

2 Samuel 12:21-22 (NIV)

21 His attendants asked him, "Why are you acting this way? While the child was alive, you fasted and wept, but now that the child is dead, you get up and eat!"

22 He answered, "While the child was still alive, I fasted and wept. I thought, 'Who knows? The Lord may be gracious to me and let the child live.'

I learn so much from David's behavior here. He was going to fast and do everything he could to save his child, but once it was over, he got up and ate. I think that time of fasting prepared him for what was coming. He left the results in God's hands. The fast did not save his son, but it prepared him for the loss of his son. At this time, my fasting has not brought my Nan into a personal walk with God, but it has given me peace in the meantime in knowing that I am doing everything I can, and it is in God's hands now. Fasting either changes your circumstance or prepares you to handle the circumstance.

Fasting is not a magic wishing well to get what you want from God. Last year, I fasted for 36-hours before speaking at a real estate conference. I fasted for clarity to hear from God and to have a powerful time. The conference went really well! The following day, I held a book signing and during my fast I prayed for that too. I wanted it to go quickly so that my friend, who had traveled with me, and I could enjoy the rest of the day together. So, I prayed I would sell out of books fast. Once I got to the Barnes & Noble where we were hosting the signing, I realized very quickly that that wasn't going to happen. There wasn't a soul there. Even the employee that worked there said it was their slowest Saturday in a while.

I didn't stress it for a second. I left books with the employee to give away to anyone who might show up and left to enjoy the rest of my day. My friend and I laughed about it and kept a positive attitude. I even walked up to random people throughout the day and gave them my books as the Lord led me. Did everything turn out the way I prayed? No, but my fasting prepared me for what did happen and I didn't lose an ounce of sleep over it.

When Jesus prayed in the Garden of Gethsemane, He didn't want to go to the cross, but He put God's will above His own. That put His heart where it needed to be to get Him through His passion.

Sometimes people will pray and fast for things because they think it will make God answer their prayers with a "yes." That's not always the case. Fasting doesn't automatically solve every problem the way you want.

Proverbs 2:8 (NIV)

"for he guards the course of the just and protects

the way of his faithful ones."

Sometimes God says no to protect you even if it doesn't look like protection at first. Remember when the king was going to throw Daniel into the lions' den? I can imagine Daniel praying to not be thrown in, but instead God shut the lions' mouths. It was a better miracle! It was the same thing with Shadrach, Meshach, and Abednego. Instead of saving them from being tossed into the fire, God had them come through it without being burned. Sometimes, we may have to go through the hard time, but God protects us in the end.

Paul was in jail when I'm sure he would have rather been out preaching, but while he was there he wrote so many books of the New Testament. God had a bigger vision.

Reasons God Says No:

1. He has a better vision for you.
2. He has a better solution.
3. So you can help other people with your problem.

One of my favorite songs is "Unanswered Prayers" by Garth Brooks. In one of the verses, he describes meeting an old high school flame while attending a football game with his wife. He thinks back to when he used to pray that God would give him that girl to marry, and realizes that one of God's greatest gifts to him was an unanswered prayer.

Isaiah 55:8 (NIV)

"For my thoughts are not your thoughts,

neither are your ways my ways,"

declares the Lord.

Sometimes our ways don't match God's ways. Sometimes the issues we're asking God to fix are problems we brought on ourselves, yet we want Him to fix it our way. You can expect a "no" if you ask God to get out of debt by helping you win at poker in Vegas. Liposuction might be the fastest way to lose weight, but that might not be God's way if you have a problem with overeating.

There are people in the Bible who didn't get exactly what they wanted. David wanted to build the temple, but God said no, so He let him do other things to prepare for it. In the end, God wanted Solomon to do it.

Moses never got to go to the Promised Land. There are some things we don't understand and other things won't get fulfilled until we get to Heaven to be with Jesus.

Before I moved into the house I live in now, I was very interested in a bank foreclosure that I thought was perfect for me. I wrote a contract on it and spent six months trying to get that house before the whole deal fell apart. I was so upset at God about that. However, six months later I found the house I live in now. It's almost three times bigger, sits on the water, and has a better floor plan. We even got millions of dollars worth of equity the day we moved in. I live within walking distance of that other house and whenever I see it I think about "Unanswered Prayers". I begged God for that house, but he didn't give it to me, and I'm grateful. I had a plan, but God had something better for me. I believe God had me tied up with that other house for six months so I could wait for this one.

I've asked God to remove my struggle with eating, but I finally realized that without these struggles I wouldn't be able to minister to other people with the books I've written. I may always have a thyroid issue. I've struggled with thyroid problems, candida, and psoriasis off and on for years. There have been times when it's gotten better and times when it's gotten worse. I prayed over and over again for God to take it away, but it kept recurring. However, I've come to realize something. Don't waste your pain and hardship that you can use to help other people.

Psalm 25:10 (NIV)

All the ways of the Lord are loving and faithful toward those who keep the demands of his covenant.

Romans 8:28 (NIV)

And we know that in all things God works for the good of those who love him, who have been called according to his purpose.

As soon as God says "no", the Devil will try to tell you that God doesn't love you. There are tons of times when I started doubting myself because of my health problems. Satan would plant an idea that God didn't love me because of what I had to deal with. God's "no" is motivated by love. Instead of getting angry like a child, pray and ask God for strength to not sink into those feelings.

Luke 22:42 (NIV)

[42] "Father, if you are willing, take this cup from me; yet not my will, but yours be done."

Chapter 11
PRAYER

One of the things I have a really hard time with is concentration. This is no different when it comes to praying. I find it so hard to stay focused while I am praying that I had to come up with a way to be able to focus on what I want to say. I have started to write out my prayers in a journal. While this isn't for everyone, since some people can stay focused and not have to worry about, it has been essential for me. What I do with my journal is write down my prayers before I say them. This helps me stay intentional and on topic with my prayers and avoid getting distracted. In the story of David and the lion's den from the Bible that we previously talked about, I use the way David prayed as an example in my daily life. David went by his open window and he went ahead and prayed to God three times a day, every day. I love the focus that David had and his commitment to prayer. With me, I have found that I start praying and all the sudden I'll start thinking, "Did my assistant do this? Was that trip planned? What is going on at work?", and the list goes on and on. I start thinking about every other thing going on in my mind no matter what it is. To help myself, in conjunction with journaling my prayers, I've also started utilizing a formula that I made. I love a good acronym and knew I had to come up with one to utilize during my prayer time. PATOM is the acronym I came up with in regards to my prayer time.

PATOM broken down stands for:

P- Praise

Admit Sins

T- Thank God

O- Pray for Other People

M- Pray for Me

The first thing is to start with praise and admiration, thanking God for who he is and how amazing of a King He is. Next is to admit your sins and confess to God, asking for forgiveness. The third step in my prayer routine is to thank God for anything and everything. The "O" in PATOM stands for praying for other people. It is important to keep others in mind and pray specific prayers for them. You may know what to pray for through conversation and community with others by asking God to put certain things on your heart for others. Lastly, I pray for myself and the things that I need. As I said earlier, I tend to write down my prayers and then speak them to God. This is helpful and keeps me focused, but it also is a really great thing to look back on. I love that when I write the prayers down, I can go back and look at them at a later time. Sometimes I'll think, "I can't believe I prayed for that or was worried about that," and it is a really powerful thing to be able to look back and see how God has answered prayers and to see the results.

The thing about prayer that is so important is that it needs to be done to the glory of God. Once I go through the steps of PATOM, I feel that my faith tank starts to fill up. I find that sometimes before prayer I may be uneasy or unsure, but by the end, I find myself always saying, "Of course you can handle this, God." In 2 Kings 19:19 (NIV), Hezekiah has a prayer that says, "Deliver us from your hands so that all the kingdoms on Earth will know that you alone are God." This is one of the most important things we need to add to our prayers. We need to be sure that we pray so that God can be glorified by whatever it is we are praying for. We need to pray for ourselves and others and the things we need, but also not forget to pray for God's glory to come out of whatever it is we're praying for. A lot of the time, if you look in scripture at different people's prayers, it will end with the words, "so that you can be glorified." They're not asking for God to deliver them from what they're facing so that they can keep their job or make more money. When people in scripture pray, they are asking to be delivered from certain things so that Christ can be glorified. The two words that stand out most to me from this specific verse are the words "so that". The prayers are being prayed so that God will be glorified through them. Whatever you want or are praying for, it needs to be for His glory. That needs to be the reason why we want what we pray for. I memorized the entire book of James, and the verse here that sticks out to me in regards to prayer is in James 4:3 (NIV). This verse says, "When you ask, you do not receive, because you ask with wrong motives, that you may spend what you get on your pleasures."

God is not our genie that is just going to give us every little thing we want.

He wants to answer our prayers so that He can be glorified through them. We need to add this request to the end of every prayer. We need to pray that everyone can come to know God, and that God can be glorified through what He does for us. We need to pray that so everyone will know that God is the Lord of Lords and King of Kings. Whatever the "so that" is for you and for your prayer, it has to be so that you can give Him the glory. He doesn't do these things for you to get glory for yourself. His chief priority is that he wants to make things so that everyone comes to know Him. I just love that verse from 2 Kings 19:19 (NIV) so much. The prayer that everyone on Earth will know that God alone is the Lord our God. This is so that all kingdoms would fall on their knees and worship God. That is the best filter you can add to the end of your prayers. Anytime I ask God to intervene in my life through prayer, I ask myself why I want whatever it is I'm asking for. For example, why do I want this commercial building that I'm looking for? Is it just another prayer that I want so that my life can become easier or be more "cushy"? Is there any glory that God can get from this want? I need to put it in my mind that what I do is for God's glory. I need to put it in my mind that I pray so that people will come to know God and will lift Him up. In doing this, you can then pray with enormous faith and confidence. I need to know that my sole purpose for the prayer that I'm praying is that God will be glorified. Instead of being selfish and praying for what is all about me, I have to keep this my priority. You have to ask yourself that question. Are you putting God's glory at the forefront of your prayers? If you are able to do that, you will pray with enormous faith and confidence.

GOD'S ANSWERS TO PRAYER

God answers every prayer, but He doesn't always say, "yes." Sometimes it's an obvious "yes", however other times it's a "no" or "not right now." One thing God will never do is give you something that will harm you. Sometimes, we pray for things that aren't helpful to us. If that's the case, He won't give it to you. He knows what we need better than we do.

Matthew 7:9-12 (NIV)

[9] **"Which of you, if your son asks for bread, will give him a stone?** [10] **Or if he asks for a fish, will give him a snake?** [11] **If you, then, though you are evil, know how to give good gifts to your children, how much more will your Father in heaven give good gifts to those who ask him!** [12] **So in everything, do to others what you would have them do to you, for this sums up the Law and the Prophets.**

From this scripture we see that if you ask God for something good, He's not going to give you something bad. He's going to give you something good. That means that if you ask for something bad, He's not going to give you that either! I remember one time my son, Kyle, asked for "a really sharp knife so I can open this box." Obviously, I didn't give it to him because I knew he could get injured if I gave it to him. God is the same way. He's a loving God and He's going to give you what's best for you.

Imagine you interview for a job that you really want. You beg God for it, but you don't get it. Here's the thing: you don't know what that job is really like. It could be terrible. Your would-be co-workers could be impossible to work with. You may want the job, but that doesn't mean it's good for you. God knows the things you don't know. When He says, "no," it's for your own good. Be conscious of this when you feel like there are doors being shut in your face over and over again. I felt like I was dealing with a closed door when it came to my struggle with weight loss. I kept asking God to take it from me so I didn't have to deal with it anymore. However, because of my struggle, I've been able to write a book and help other people with similar problems as me. In the end, it's been a blessing.

At the same time, God is not a "Santa Claus" God. He's not a slot machine to get what you want out of Him. He's not a genie in the bottle, but HE IS your Father who gives good gifts to you.

PERSISTENCE IN PRAYER

Let's talk about praying during a fast. When I was in high school, I memorized the entire book of James. It was part of the Bible study I was in, and we ended up going to California for a trip, and one of the things that they required us to do for this trip was to memorize this book. There's one portion in particular that I want to go over and share with you.

James 4:1-4 (NIV)

"What causes fights and quarrels among you?

Don't they come from your desires that battle

within you? You desire but you do not have, so you

kill. You covet but you cannot get what you want, so

you quarrel and fight. You do not have because you

do not ask God. When you ask, you do not receive,

because you ask with wrong motives, that you may

spend what you get on your pleasures."

In this passage, James gives two reasons behind why our prayers don't get answered. The first is that we simply don't ask for it. The second is that we do ask, but with the wrong motives. We are asking God to do something for us, but it is really for us to have more comfort, not to better His kingdom.

Colossians 4:2 (NIV)

² Devote yourselves to prayer, being watchful and

thankful.

Why do I have to pray for something more than one time? Is it because God wants you to keep begging Him? Does He need you to pester Him? Is He going to say, "Enough already! Stop asking!" No, that's not the God we serve.

There are two types of parables in the Bible, comparing parables and contrasting parables. Comparing parables show you what God is like and contrasting parables show you something that's in contrast to Him. We're going to look at two contrasting parables.

Luke 11:5-9 (NIV)

[5] Then Jesus said to them, "Suppose you have a friend, and you go to him at midnight and say, 'Friend, lend me three loaves of bread; [6] a friend of mine on a journey has come to me, and I have no food to offer him.' [7] And suppose the one inside answers, 'Don't bother me. The door is already locked, and my children and I are in bed. I can't get up and give you anything.' [8] I tell you, even though he will not get up and give you the bread because of friendship, yet because of your shameless audacity he will surely get up and give you as much as you need.

[9] "So I say to you: Ask and it will be given to you; seek and you will find; knock and the door will be opened to you.

My neighbors and I are the best of friends. Our sons hang out together all the time and our families get together for cookouts. We get along great! However, as close as we are, waking them up in the middle of a night for three loaves of bread would be a bit much! If you're persistent, though, people will give in to what you want. Jesus used this parable to illustrate how we should be persistent in prayer. The neighbor is a contrast to God, but Jesus wants us to be persistent and ask for things more than once.

Luke 18:2-8 (NIV)

² He said: "In a certain town there was a judge who neither feared God nor cared what people thought.

³ And there was a widow in that town who kept coming to him with the plea, 'Grant me justice against my adversary.'

⁴ "For some time he refused. But finally he said to himself, 'Even though I don't fear God or care what people think, ⁵ yet because this widow keeps bothering me, I will see that she gets justice, so that she won't eventually come and attack me!'"

⁶ And the Lord said, "Listen to what the unjust judge says. ⁷ And will not God bring about justice for his chosen ones, who cry out to him day and night? Will he keep putting them off? ⁸ I tell you, he will see that they get justice, and quickly. However, when the Son of Man comes, will he find faith on the earth?"

If you're feeling discouraged, that means you should be praying. If you're not praying, that means you've given up! Ask yourself if you stopped praying persistently. Have you given up? Sometimes the answer isn't a "no," it's just a "not now." So, keep asking. It's not about convincing God.

Let's say you have a drinking problem you can't beat. You ask God to take it away, but He hasn't. Why not? When you have an issue, your attention is on God, which is where He wants it. In fact, you spend the most time with God when you have a problem. When everything is fine, you spend less time with Him. So, I'm continually looking to God for help. God wants us to go to Him for strength.

2 Corinthians 12:10 (NIV)

¹⁰ That is why, for Christ's sake, I delight in weaknesses, in insults, in hardships, in persecutions, in difficulties. For when I am weak, then I am strong.

While you're praying for an answer, you're going to learn more than you would any other way. You're going to learn more about yourself when you don't get everything you want right away. There are some things I've prayed about that God has answered right away. There are other things that took a long time.

Just remember that there isn't anybody who doesn't have a laundry list of issues. Don't be fooled by the glamour you see on Facebook.

Thank God!

Thank God in advance for answered prayer.

2 Chronicles 20:21-23 (NIV)

²¹ After consulting the people, Jehoshaphat appointed men to sing to the Lord and to praise him for the splendor of his holiness as they went out at the head of the army, saying:

"Give thanks to the Lord,

for his love endures forever."

²² As they began to sing and praise, the Lord set ambushes against the men of Ammon and Moab and Mount Seir who were invading Judah, and they were defeated. ²³ The Ammonites and Moabites rose up against the men from Mount Seir to destroy and annihilate them. After they finished slaughtering the men from Seir, they helped to destroy one another.

The king wanted the singers and band singing "thank you" before they even won the battle. Thank God in advance for healing your body, taking care of your pain, and restoring your finances. See how those enemy armies started fighting each other? Judah won the battle without even lifting a finger! God turns battles into blessings! We need to start putting the choir out first. Sing praises and put on worship songs. Thank God in advance for everything He's going to do in your life. You don't have to be able to sing to do this.

2 Chronicles 20:25-26 (NIV)

²⁵ So Jehoshaphat and his men went to carry off their plunder, and they found among them a great amount of equipment and clothing and also articles of value—more than they could take away. There

was so much plunder that it took three days to collect it. ²⁶ On the fourth day they assembled in the Valley of Berakah, where they praised the Lord. This is why it is called the Valley of Berakah to this day.

It took three days to gather the spoils! On the fourth day, they assembled a worship service and named that place the Valley of Blessing - that's what "berakah" means. If you've been fighting a battle with food, drinking, your marriage, finances, or anything, sing and rejoice that God will turn it around for blessing. This passage of Scripture is one of my favorite stories. You can read to encourage yourself anytime you feel worried or afraid.

2 Chronicles 20:15-16 (NIV)

¹⁵ He said: "Listen, King Jehoshaphat and all who live in Judah and Jerusalem! This is what the Lord says to you: 'Do not be afraid or discouraged because of this vast army. For the battle is not yours, but God's. ¹⁶ Tomorrow march down against them. They will be climbing up by the Pass of Ziz, and you will find them at the end of the gorge in the Desert of Jeruel.

If you're reading this and have never given your life to Christ, now is the time. Say these words aloud:

God, I've been trying to fight on my own. Now, I want you to come in and be the pilot of my life. Come into my heart and life. I want to live for you. I don't want to keep failing with this problem over and over again. I know you died on the cross for me. I want to spend eternity with You. I know that I don't deserve it. I know there's no good amount of works that can earn my way in. I know it's the blood of Jesus - the one who died for me on the cross - covering my sins so I can spend eternity with You forever.

2 Chronicles 20:30 (NIV)

[30] And the kingdom of Jehoshaphat was at peace, for his God had given him rest on every side.

This is the breakthrough you're searching for: peace in the area of your former struggle. This is when God takes you to a whole new level.

Chapter 12
STRENGTH IN NUMBERS / HANDS RAISED UP

Exodus 17:8-16 (NIV)

8 The Amalekites came and attacked the Israelites at Rephidim. 9 Moses said to Joshua, "Choose some of our men and go out to fight the Amalekites. Tomorrow I will stand on top of the hill with the staff of God in my hands."

10 So Joshua fought the Amalekites as Moses had ordered, and Moses, Aaron, and Hur went to the top of the hill. 11 As long as Moses held up his hands, the Israelites were winning, but whenever he lowered his hands, the Amalekites were winning. 12 When Moses' hands grew tired, they took a stone and put it under him and he sat on it. Aaron and Hur held his hands up—one on one side, one on the other—so that his hands remained steady till

sunset. [13] **So Joshua overcame the Amalekite army with the sword.**

[14] **Then the LORD said to Moses, "Write this on a scroll as something to be remembered and make sure that Joshua hears it because I will completely blot out the name of Amalek from under heaven."**

[15] **Moses built an altar and called it The LORD is my Banner.** [16] **He said, "Because hands were lifted up against[a] the throne of the LORD,[b] the LORD will be at war against the Amalekites from generation to generation."**

In Exodus 17:8-15 (NIV), the story of Moses, Joshua, Aaron, and Hur is told. This story is a beautiful example of the necessity of praising God with our hands raised up, both literally and figuratively, and the importance of having a community around us. In this passage, the Israelites were being invaded by the Amalekites. Moses knew that if nothing is done, the battle would be a complete massacre. The Israelites were not prepared for battle, and if this happened, hundreds of thousands of his people would be killed. Moses knew it would be an unfair battle. However, he had three people that were his community in this – Aaron, Hur, and Joshua. They were all in their eighties, and not sure what to do at this point with the impending battle. Moses instructeds Joshua to go and round up as many men as he couldan get, so Joshua wentgoes and grabbeds some men.

At that time, Moses went up on the hill with Aaron and Hur. The men did not do anything specific to help in battle other than pray and hold their hands up high to the Lord.

This reminds of me of something my son would do when he was around two or three. My son, Kyle, would lift his hands up over his head and turn to me asking me to pick him up and hold him. This is such a natural tendency for children to do when they need comfort and their caregiver, and it is no different with God. Moses made the decision to do the only thing he could do, which was lift his arms up high to God. He did what believers should do in a situation in which we don't know what else to do. I imagine Moses thinking, "I need supernatural help. I don't know what to do. I've got this huge army facing me, and I need you, God." In Exodus 17:11 (NIV) it says, "as long as Moses held up his hands, the Israelites were winning, but whenever he lowered his hands, the Amalekites were winning." Moses raising his hands up to the Lord was the only thing keeping the Israelites alive and winning the battle.

There is something in every person's life that causes them to feel so overwhelmed and so exhausted that they don't know what to do. There are daily battles that each one of us face, and these battles are different for each one of us. A lot of times, when we really need God's guidance, is when we instead start turning to other things such as food, drugs, alcohol, or shopping. Everyone has a vice that is easy to turn to when we don't know what else to do. We run to these things such as an activity or food because we are so sad or depressed that we lack the energy to make better choices. Let's look back at the significance of the hands raised above Moses's head. I wonder how long it took him, Aaron and Hur to realize that his hands being in the air affected the outcome of the battle. They might have realized that the reason he put his hands down was because he was tired. However, the Bible doesn't say how long it took them to realize that when his hands were up, they were winning, and when they were down, they were not.

There is a big connection between us and our troubles based on the times when our hands are up in the air and the times when they are brought down. When they are raised up to the Lord, is when we are winning our personal battle. However, as soon as we get tired and we bring them down, we may begin to lose. This is exactly what was happening with Moses during this battle. In this case, it was a one to one correspondence between the location of his hands and the outcome of the battle. I really want the imagery of what this means to stick with you as you read this story. We want to be thinking about it over and over again. I want us to fully think and understand how when our arms are in the air, raised up to Him, God is with us.

One of the things that would be helpful to do as a real-life example is to have two people sit on the couch next to you and sing a worship song. Put your hands in the air and sing this worship song while keeping your arms in the air for as long as you can. With your friends sitting next to you, see how long you can do this. When you start getting tired and you just can't keep your arms lifted, sing another song. During this song, have your friends next to you try and help you to hold them up. There have been times in my life when my arms have been raised during a really hard time. However, there were other times where I got defeated and I brought my hands down. This is why it's so important to have people right next to you being your Aaron and your Hur. Who are those people in your life? Ask yourself if you have people in your life that when your arms start moving down, you know that they are there to help you keep them up. If you don't, you need to pray and ask God to bring these people into your life to hold your hands up when you can no longer do it by yourself anymore. This needs to be a conversation between you and God.

Think about some times in your life when you have actually lifted your hands up and felt like you were winning a battle. Now, think about other times when your arms were low and things were hard, and you felt like you were losing the battle you were facing. In your mind, you have to be conscious about where the locations of your hands are, especially during the tough times. If raised hands can help you win the battle, why do we ever lower them? When Moses' hands were tired (which is a normal thing, remember that he was 80!), he had Aaron and Hur next to him to give him encouragement and prayer and help him to keep his arms raised. There are times in all of our lives when we might get discouraged and find ourselves defeated and without prayer. Maybe these feelings happened because you feel like you've prayed about the same thing over and over again. Maybe you got to the point where you feel like Paul and feel like you have a thorn in your side that is just not going to go away. For me, there are a couple of times I can think about when I feel like I have lowered my hands. One of these times that comes to mind is in regards to my hunt for a perfect location for our corporate office. My dream would be to find a building that a church could use on the weekend to hold their services. For whatever reason, I have not been able to buy a property even though I have been saving money and constantly looking and praying. For some reason, nothing has opened up yet.

It is easy to get discouraged when you have prayed and prayed about something and finally realize that it maybe isn't what God wants. People will ask me if I've prayed about this scenario, and it would be easy to get nasty since it is something that I have obviously done. The ugly truth is that sometimes your hands get tired, and sometimes your faith dies, and sometimes the hope of things goes away. Sometimes the hope you have has gotten bashed so many times that just when you think something is going to happen and it doesn't, your hope continues to get deflated. This same thing may happen when it comes to your eating. Maybe you've lost weight and think things are going really well and then it turns around and goes the opposite direction. You are not the only person that has a certain area in their life that you feel like you've been praying about over and over again, so try not to feel alone. We all have our battles with this.

One other area that I notice this in my life is regarding my grandmother. I've prayed and prayed over and over again for her to give her life to Christ. For years, there has been no answer. Sometimes, there are just mysteries of unanswered prayers in our lives. We have to continue to look at what happens when our hands get tired. One thing Moses did in this story was put a stone underneath him to sit on. Then, Aaron and Hur, his brother and brother-in-law, came, held his hands, and remained with him, praying until sunset. Because of this, Joshua overcame the Amalekite army. After winning the battle, Joshua came to tell Moses that they were in this with him all along and that he was not alone. Aaron and Hur had promised to stay with Moses and keep his arms up for however long it took. These are what I call "arm lifters." When you have a really big prayer request, you need some arm lifters on your side.

During the times when your faith tank may be dried out, you need others to pour some of their faith into your tank. We all have times when we feel our tank emptying, and it's important to put our trust into others and God to help us fill it back up. When you feel them pouring some of their faith into your tank, it makes such a big difference. These are the times when you need to cry out and thank God that you have these people in your life who can encourage you and pray with and over you. If you do not feel this way, you need to ask God to bring you an Aaron and a Hur. This has become one of my favorite stories in the Bible that I can directly apply to my life. The image of the arm lifters is one that stays with me. Ask yourself if this is happening in your life, and if you have these types of people you can rely on. These things don't happen without being in community or Bible study. On the opposite end, there also might be a Moses in your life that you could be a blessing for to help lift their arms up. Sometimes you are Moses, and sometimes you are Aaron and Hur. It is so important to pray and see who God directs you to that might need the help from you. There might be some people that are struggling in their health, marriage, or family, amongst other things, but you don't learn these things if you are not in a small and honest community.

When I think about this story, that Aaron and Hur held up Moses's arms until sunset, I couldn't help but think how long of a time that had to have been. These three older men put time on the backburner to encourage and support their friend and brother while trusting and praising God. They stayed that way for hours and hours and hours. This makes me think about the times when I feel like I just don't have time for even a 5-minute prayer. It is so important to put aside the time to raise our hands to the Lord and spend time in prayer with Him. After the battle, the Lord instructed Moses to write what had happened so that it would always be remembered. This was God telling Moses that this analogy of the raised hands and the story in its entirety was something that should be remembered. He wanted to make sure that Moses and everyone else remembered what had been done. It is so important for us to remember this in our daily life as well. Are we constantly reminding ourselves about the position of our hands? Let's make this a priority, and keep our hands raised up to the Lord.

PART 4

Hope Acronym

Chapter 13
FASTING TO HEAR AND HEAL

PART 1: FASTING TO HEAR

One of my favorite passages in the Bible is a story of a young man named Samuel. He was ministering with an old man named Eli, and they both lived at the church from what I understand. Samuel kept interrupting the sleep of Eli, saying that he kept hearing from someone, and every time he heard he would say "Here I am," thinking it was Eli calling him. Samuel didn't realize that it was God calling him, not Eli. So finally Eli said to Samuel "Next time you hear the voice, say 'Speak Lord, your servant is listening.'"

I relate to this story because sometimes when God speaks to me, I get confused. I can think I am hearing from someone else besides God. It can be hard to tell if it's really him!

One night I was sleeping in bed, and I felt like God was telling me to go check and see if I had closed the garage door. I knew that I had closed the garage door! But God kept telling me to go check. Finally, I couldn't sleep, so I went downstairs and the door was indeed closed! I was like, "What in the world, God, I was trying to sleep," and I felt I heard Him saying "I just wanted to make sure you were listening." I receive prompts all the time. Sometimes the prompts don't go anywhere, but most of the time they do.

When I meet people, I always ask what they eat for breakfast, lunch and dinner. I've interview over 1,000 people over the past 20 years. Back in the beginning of this, maybe 18 years ago, God prompted me to go to my aerobics teacher and ask her what she had for breakfast! We've remained friends and I have planted seeds by inviting her to church, although she didn't want to come, encouraging her, and sending her messages to listen to online. Planting seeds over and over again. I will send Christian podcasts, Christian songs, or anything I think might speak to her.

About a year ago, God prompted me to randomly invite her over to the house. It was a really loud prompt. I had purchased this movie called "The Case for Christ," and God told me he wanted me to invite Jenn and Willy to have dinner and watch the movie. After they watched the movie, a couple of days later, Jenn told me that she and her husband both wanted to give their lives to Christ. About a week and a half later, I baptized their entire family in my pool! One of the things they said is that all of the things I had sent them over the years got them to a place where they were ready to receive Christ. Those were all little prompts God gave me; I was listening to a song and God said "Send this to Jenn and Willy," listening to a sermon and He said, "Send this to Jenn and Willy." Now their entire family has given their lives to Christ! A lot of people, after 18 years of friendship, would have given up, but I continued to obey the whispers of God.

Going back to Samuel, a prayer we should be praying every day is, "Give me Samuel's ear to hear every whisper of you." It's not just about listening, it's obeying what He tells you to do. I always seek to listen and obey, and I am blown away by what God does.

While you fast, you need to urgently pray that God will allow you to hear his voice loud and clear like Samuel did. In this chapter, we are going to learn how to recognize and decipher the voice of God.

Acts 18:21 (NIV)

21 But as he left, he promised, "I will come back if it

is God's will." Then he set sail from Ephesus.

I used to know a person who always ended statements with "Lord willing" no matter what the conversation was about. If she was leaving for the grocery store, she would say, "I'll see you in a little while, Lord willing." Or if you asked what she would like to eat she might respond, "I would love to have lasagna for dinner, Lord willing." After a while it got annoying to hear that all the time. One day, I asked her why she kept saying that and she read me this scripture:

James 4:15 (NIV)

15 Instead, you ought to say, "If it is the Lord's will,

we will live and do this or that."

Now, if you look at this with the lens of Biblical truth, technically you wouldn't add this caveat to every statement, but it rubbed off on me and I say it now, too.

Proverbs 16:9 (NIV)

⁹ In their hearts humans plan their course,

but the Lord establishes their steps.

Learning to decipher if it is God's voice you are hearing, or someone else is so important! Make sure that whatever you're doing, it's the will of God. Use the VOICE system (below) whenever you're confronted with a decision you're not sure about. Run the decision through these checkpoints to determine if the choice you're making is in line with God's will:

V- Vocalize- Talk to your Godly friends.

O- Open Doors- Are doors opening or closing?

I- Is this Biblical? - Does the decision line up with God's Word?

C- Confirmation of the Holy Spirit- Ask Him for peace in the decision.

E- Emulate Your Talents- Does this match your talents?

This system will work no matter how confused or unsettled you are. Challenge your situation with these questions to see if it passes the test. These are your checkpoints before you say, "YES." I'll elaborate more below.

1) **V- Vocalize-** Talk to your Godly friends.

Proverbs 11:14 (NIV)

¹⁴ For lack of guidance a nation falls,

but victory is won through many advisers.

Proverbs 20:18 (NIV)

[18] Plans are established by seeking advice;

so if you wage war, obtain guidance.

Bring your decision under the scrutiny of godly friends you trust. What do I mean by godly? I'm talking about Christians who spend time in the Word daily, go to church, love God, and have a fellowship with Him. No one is flawless, but you should be seeking the advice of people who are a good reflection of honoring Christ. Those people for me are my husband, pastor, mother, sister, and a couple of my friends. These are people who I know I need to listen to when they tell me something.

One point I want to make now and that I'll make again is that you can't depend on only one of the letters of VOICE. All of the checkpoints have to work together or you'll still miss the will of God. When you're seeking advice from godly friends, the advice still has to match the Word of God (letter I). You have to be careful of that because you can get good advice from ten different godly people but they can all point you in a different direction. Before I got into real estate, I sought out godly advice. While most of the people I talked to encouraged me to follow this new path I believed God was setting me on, a few told me not to go. Thankfully, I made the right decision and the rest is history!

2) O- Open Doors- Are doors opening or closing?

Suppose there's a job that you're convinced God wants you to have, but they won't hire you. That would be a door closing. It is important to recognize how what we want can sometimes be different than what God wants for us.

Revelation 3:8 (NIV)

8 ··· See, I have placed before you an open door that no one can shut ...

Not only does God open doors no man can shut, he also shuts doors no man can open. God can use circumstances to lead and guide us.

Acts 16:7-10 (NIV)

7 When they came to the border of Mysia, they tried to enter Bithynia, but the Spirit of Jesus would not allow them to. 8 So they passed by Mysia and went down to Troas. 9 During the night Paul had a vision of a man of Macedonia standing and begging him, "Come over to Macedonia and help us." 10 After Paul had seen the vision, we got ready at once to leave for Macedonia, concluding that God had called us to preach the gospel to them.

This passage is from Paul's second missionary journey. He wanted to go one way, but the Spirit of God said no and he had to go another direction. Paul saw how God was working in his circumstances. God shut different doors and Paul concluded that God had to be sending him to Macedonia.

Let's dig deeper into the story of how I got into real estate, as an example. I had been working as a children's pastor up to that point, but I was burnt out from the ministry. There were all kinds of things happening to the point that I was beginning to hate the ministry. I felt like God was telling me to go into ministry in the marketplace so I prayed about real estate. I took the real estate license test and passed in a week. It was so easy for me. After that, a lady at my church invited me to work with her at the agency where she was an agent. It worked out perfectly. Every door opened up without a struggle.

One of my friends, Dana, told me she wanted to quit her job as a keyboarding teacher to be a motivational speaker on entrepreneurship. She asked for my advice on what to do and I told her to start doing her motivational talks at night and on weekends so she could still support her family with her job and test it out to see what doors were opening or closing. This made sense for her to practically see where God was leading her without immediately diving in.

3) I-Is this Biblical? Does the decision line up with God's Word?

Ask yourself this: does this decision jive with the character of God? Did this idea come from God or is it something I came up with myself? One time, I had a friend of mine give me a prophetic word from God. He said that God was going to bless me soon in a powerful way but that I had to make sure I gave all the glory to Him.

After he told me this, I thought, "I don't know if he heard from God or not, but I know that what He said aligns with the Word." There are tons of verses on giving God the glory and not yourself. Whether or not the prophecy was from God (and I'm sure it was), it was something that lined up with Scripture. When you receive a prompting from God directly or through someone else, bump it up against God's character.

One aspect of God's character is wisdom, so you should always ask yourself if the decision you're about to make is wise.

I run into people all the time who stop using wisdom when they're buying a house. They find a house they love that's $50,000 higher than their budget. It gets worse when the market is hot because you have to make a decision right away if you don't want to lose a house. Godly wisdom says to stick to your budget no matter what's going on.

How about wisdom in relationships? Say that you meet someone and you're both ready to get married after two weeks. Why don't you slow down and figure out what's going on, first? Moving that fast isn't wise.

There are many churches in the world that try to keep their "sheep under control" with legalism. So, many people avoid church because of the list of things they can't do. There are churches full of people living in bondage when we have freedom in Christ.

I experienced this kind of freedom many years ago when I attended what was at the time the first church I'd been to in a long time. The pastor there asked if I wanted to join his small group and I told him I would as long as he didn't have a problem with me smoking with no plans to quit. He told me they loved people as they were and invited me to come. A few months after I joined that Bible study group, I quit smoking. Nobody asked me to. It was what I was compelled to do after coming closer to God and learning my body was a temple.

So, how do you decide whether you should or shouldn't do something? I like to use the example of a filter. I make my own almond milk, and when I blend almonds in my Vitamix, I pour the milk into a nutbag. It's a filter that stops everything that's not milk. It's a filter. You should have a filter, too. If any action or decision is going to cause stoppage in your life, then it's something you shouldn't do. If it doesn't pass through the filter, then it shouldn't be in your life.

First, determine if the Bible strictly prohibits something. If so, it's obviously something you shouldn't do. That can mean anything from adultery, murder, and stealing to breaking your word, overeating, and lying. However, not everything appears so black and white.

1 Corinthians 10:23 (NIV)

23 "I have the right to do anything," you say—but not everything is beneficial. "I have the right to do anything"—but not everything is constructive.

There are some things we can do without losing God's love or favor, but this doesn't mean we should.

1 Peter 1:16 (NIV)

[16] for it is written: "Be holy, because I am holy."

Second, ask if what you're doing will harm you physically. If so, you're damaging God's property.

1 Corinthians 6:19-20 (NIV)

[19] Do you not know that your bodies are temples of the Holy Spirit, who is in you, whom you have received from God? You are not your own; 20 you were bought at a price. Therefore honor God with your bodies.

We want to honor God with our bodies. Think about what you eat. Is it hurting or healing your body? It's not your property to hurt. Think about it: when you're staying in someone else's home, you take really good care of their stuff even more than you would your own possessions. That's what it's like.

Some things are much easier to judge because they blatantly defy God's Word. Here are some quick and easy ones.

- Should I have sex with my boyfriend? **1 Corinthians 6:18 (NIV) - Flee from sexual immorality …**

- Is God telling me to marry him/her even though they're not saved? **2 Corinthians 6:14 (NIV) - Do not be yoked together with unbelievers …**

- Do I have to report my income on my taxes? **Exodus 20:15 (NIV) - "You shall not steal. Matthew 22:21 (NIV) - … Then he said to them, "So give back to Caesar what is Caesar's …**

- I want to get back at the person who hurt me. **Romans 12:19 (NIV) - Do not take revenge, my dear friends, but leave room for God's wrath, for it is written: "It is mine to avenge; I will repay," says the Lord.**

- Should I cheat on my spouse? **Exodus 20:14 (NIV) - "You shall not commit adultery. Hebrews 13:4 (NIV) - Marriage should be honored by all, and the marriage bed kept pure, for God will judge the adulterer and all the sexually immoral.**

- Should I eat this entire pie by myself? **Proverbs 23:2 (NIV) - and put a knife to your throat if you are given to gluttony.**

- Should I quit my job even though I have kids to support? **1 Timothy 5:8 (NIV) - Anyone who does not provide for their relatives, and especially for their own household, has denied the faith and is worse than an unbeliever.**

- Should I cash out my savings to participate in a get rich quick scheme? **Proverbs 13:11 (NIV) - Dishonest money dwindles away, but whoever gathers money little by little makes it grow.**

God does not lead people contrary to His Word. If you're being tempted to make wrong decisions, that prompting did not come from God. It might have been the Devil or your own flesh, but God never leads anyone contrary to His Word.

4) C - Confirmation of the Holy Spirit- Ask Him for peace in the decision.

God is interested in life's little details. If you think you can only approach Him about big problems in your life, then you're missing out on a personal connection with Him. God is concerned about even the smallest detail. Because I know this, I pray about the things that people find silly like parking spaces and clothing sales. I act like God is my very best friend and I talk to Him about everything. Find out God's will for specific issues in your life.

Isaiah 30:21 (NIV)

21 Whether you turn to the right or to the left, your ears will hear a voice behind you, saying, "This is the way; walk in it."

John 10:27 (NIV)

27 My sheep listen to my voice; I know them, and they follow me.

The Bible doesn't talk about every issue we confront in life specifically. There's no verse in the Bible telling you whether or not to take that job. You have to pray about these kinds of issues so the Holy Spirit can tell you the way to go. All of these checkpoints help you to make the right conclusion. If the decision you want to make isn't verified by these five checkpoints, or if it's only verified by one of them, then it's a good indicator that it's not the right way.

1 Kings 19:11-13 (NIV)

11 The Lord said, "Go out and stand on the mountain in the presence of the Lord, for the Lord is about to pass by."

Then a great and powerful wind tore the mountains apart and shattered the rocks before

the Lord, but the Lord was not in the wind. After the wind there was an earthquake, but the Lord was not in the earthquake.[12] After the earthquake came a fire, but the Lord was not in the fire. And after the fire came a gentle whisper. [13] When Elijah heard it, he pulled his cloak over his face and went out and stood at the mouth of the cave.

Then a voice said to him, "What are you doing here, Elijah?"

Elijah learned to listen to the gentle whisper of God. This only happens for you when you're praying, fasting, and studying the Word regularly. You have to be seeking God on purpose. Our world gets so busy, but when we let it get too busy and too "loud", we miss out on hearing God speak to us.

Don't make a decision without peace from the Holy Spirit. However, learn to tell the difference between what you want and what the Holy Spirit says because it's easy to conjure up a sense of peace for something you badly want to do.

How do you tell the difference between the desires of your own flesh and the will of the Holy Spirit? The ability to sift through that comes from spending time with God and fasting. Fasting is that missing piece of the puzzle. You can discern more clearly when you combine fasting with your prayer.

In real estate, we often do a "pop by" with potential clients - we deliver gifts to people who are thinking about selling their homes. Christians often don't give God more than a pop by in the morning. They say a short prayer once a day and keep it moving. It's when you fast that you gain an ability to hear God's voice clearly.

A friend of mine, Sherri, and her husband moved constantly and she didn't want to the last time. She prayed for confirmation so she could have peace about moving. She decided that if the house sold immediately then it was the will of God. They put the house up for sale by owner at a time when the market wasn't hot. They had a contract the very first day. She got her confirmation.

Don't let peace be your only checkpoint. Otherwise, you'll create your own sense of peace to justify a bad decision. Here's an example: I want a new car. I don't need a new car. I want one. Since I really want one, it's easy for me to drum up a sense of peace about making that decision. That's why peace can't be the only checkpoint. You have to incorporate all of these other checkpoints as well. So, I asked my husband what he thought about me getting a new car. He said, "I think you getting a new car is fine, but we should pay off our house before you do that." He was right. That's godly wisdom. Even the Bible says that I should pay off debt.

5) E- Emulate Your Talents- Does this match your talents?

Jordan, my brother-in-law, approached me one day with an idea he had been tossing around: he was thinking about getting into real estate. "I don't think you have a gift for sales," I told him.

It was true. He wasn't a sales guy. Before you make an occupational change, ask yourself if it lines up with what God has gifted you. I would never consider getting an administrative job because I am not detailed AT ALL. However, when I first considered getting into real estate, people told me I could sell ice to an Eskimo. It was something that lined up with my gifts!

Here's the biggest thing to remember when using VOICE: you can't just pick and choose one of the letters to follow. It's all of these pieces together that lead to a right decision.

Not only when you fast are you able to hear from God, but you are also able to hear from others in a way that you never have before. I am currently fasting, and I listened to a podcast from Craig Groeschel. He said "in a work relationship, it's important to give and receive feedback from your teammates." If you have a team of five year olds playing sports, you are going to have one mom or dad coaching all the players. But once you get to a professional football team, like the Redskins, my favorite team, you have an offensive line coach, defensive line coach, head coach, and trainers. When you get in the pros, you need more specialized coaching. So if you are coaching someone, it's not because they are not good. It's because you really value them and want them to be better.

We have someone in our organization who really opposes change. When you have someone who is a wounded animal, they either retreat or attack when they feel attacked. People, like wounded animals, can retreat or attack. This particular individual, when she receives coaching or feedback, she attacks. She can't see the problem. What fasting does for you is allows you to receive feedback in a way that you can process information in a way that is helpful instead of getting defensive.

We have told this person that we feel she has anger issues, but in her mind she doesn't see them. We've offered her counseling, and she has refused that, but she has agreed to try fasting, so we are really hoping it brings that clarity. If you have people in your organization who are unwilling to receive coaching and feedback, it stifles the ability to grow. And if you cannot receive feedback, you can't grow as a person. You have to say, "I am not perfect, everyone has areas they need to work on, and if someone truly cares about me, they will give honest feedback." Fasting makes you less defensive. Think about the porcupine. Its body is covered in quills, with really sharp barbs on the end. If the porcupine is threatened, it will stick its quills out in defense and poke the attacker. Our natural reaction is to be a porcupine and stick our quills out when we get defensive, but fasting will help you to relax. Be like Samuel, not like the porcupine.

PART 2: FASTING TO HEAL

I always talk about my favorite hotel, it's the Ritz Carlton in Key Biscayne, Florida. Their customer service is over the top. At most hotels, housekeeping will come to your room once a day, if that. But at the Ritz Carlton, they come in twice! Once around 11 o'clock in the afternoon, when they make your bed, refresh your linens, pick up your trash and organize your stuff. Then, they come back again at 7 pm, to fix anything that was messed up since they last visited. They'll even give you more water bottles, turn down your bed, and put a nice chocolate on your pillow! You may be thinking, "Sounds like a great place, what does this have to do with fasting?"

Glad you asked! One of the healing benefits of fasting is autophagy, and I like to relate autophagy to housekeeping. Autophagy is your body's form of housekeeping. Not only does this burn the fat around your belly and abdominal region, which is most dangerous for heart disease, diabetes, and cancer, but it also cleans out damaged or unhealthy cells like free radicals. If you drink alcohol, it destroys tissue and leaves dead cells, autophagy will help remove these dead cells.

Really smart doctors all agree that medicine doesn't heal your body, but it aids your body in natural healing. If you want to fat-proof, disease-proof, and age-proof your body, there is nothing more beneficial than fasting.

There are so many conditions that fasting healed my body of, including my rheumatoid arthritis. My doctor once told me that my knees looked like the knees of a 70-year-old. Now, my knees are 120 times better than they were! They're not perfect, but fasting has healed the rheumatoid arthritis in my joints and muscles. Fasting also helps my psoriasis. I have polycystic ovary syndrome (PCOS) and fasting normalized my menstrual cycle. My cycles were all over the map, but now I'm at exactly 28 days. In the beginning, fasting may disrupt your cycle, but it will ultimately regulate it. Fasting slows down your aging process also, which is great for me since my husband is seven years younger than me. Medicine is great, but our bodies were designed to heal themselves, and fasting is a really key part in this.

Chapter 14
FASTING TO OVERCOME DIFFICULT TIMES

1 Corinthians 10:13 (NIV)

¹³ No temptation has overtaken you except what is common to mankind. And God is faithful; he will not let you be tempted beyond what you can bear. But when you are tempted, he will also provide a way out so that you can endure it.

There are four things to remember when getting through tough times.

1. God inspects our troubles.

If God allows a trouble in your life, you can rest assure that He has inspected it. He inspects every trial and trouble to make sure we can endure it. Whatever you're facing right now, God says, "Yes, you can endure it!" He's given you the strength to make it through.

2. There is a reason why you're going through troubles. He's going to turn it around for good.

2 Corinthians 12:7 (NKJV)

⁷ And lest I should be exalted above measure by the abundance of the revelations, a thorn in the flesh was given to me, a messenger of Satan to buffet me, lest I be exalted above measure.

Buffet translates to *kolaphizō* in Greek. It means "to strike with the *fist*; to hit hard "with the knuckles, to make the blow sting and crush (Strong's Greek). This puts me in mind of someone getting "cauliflower ear." My husband used to wrestle, so I've seen all of these wrestlers with cauliflower ear, which is an ear deformity that comes from repeated blunt force trauma. It happens when you get bashed on over and over again. Paul had a situation like that. You may have a situation that's making you feel like you're being bashed on right now. Take comfort in knowing there's a reason for it. God has seen it, planned out all the steps, and determined how it's going to end up for your good. These troubles have been calculated by God to produce character in our lives, so we can achieve what He's set out for us.

1 Thessalonians 5:18 (NIV)

¹⁸ give thanks in all circumstances; for this is God's will for you in Christ Jesus.

It's all planned as part of God's will!

3. We are not alone. God is with us!

2 Chronicles 32:6-8 (NIV)

[6] He appointed military officers over the people and assembled them before him in the square at the city gate and encouraged them with these words: [7] "Be strong and courageous. Do not be afraid or discouraged because of the king of Assyria and the vast army with him, for there is a greater power with us than with him. [8] With him is only the arm of flesh, but with us is the LORD our God to help us and to fight our battles." And the people gained confidence from what Hezekiah the king of Judah said.

In a situation that would be tough for anyone to give a pep talk about, King Hezekiah encouraged his people. The rest of the chapter details how God came through for them and delivered them.

4. God always turns our troubles around for our good like only He can do.

I like to use this visual when I am trying to encourage people at speaking engagements. It's an activity during which I ask for volunteers who like cake to come up front. However, instead of offering them cake, I bring out cake ingredients: raw eggs, flour, and oil. I get volunteers to try each ingredient. They all agree that they're disgusting and everyone gets a laugh. At the end, I bring out a delicious finished cake and make my point: life is like baking a cake. It's made up of raw and bitter ingredients that aren't enjoyable. However, God is the baker of your life and He blends the good and bad experiences together to make a good finished product.

Chapter 15

FASTING FOR PROVISION AND PROTECTION

PART 1: PROVISION

A couple years ago, I appeared on the "700 Club" where I shared my testimony about what God has taught me about giving over the years, and how He has blessed my obedience. The phone lines and email blew up at my company after the interview aired! The 700 Club said it was one of their most viewed stories. I believe this is because there are so many Christians that just can't seem to get a financial breakthrough. They find themselves in a depressing cycle of financial struggle. I truly believe that one of the reasons we are called to fast is for God's provision in this area of our lives. In Matthew 6, praying, giving, and fasting are listed as spiritual disciplines that are not optional! Let's dive in and talk about how giving and fasting are related.

Matthew 6:2, 5, 16 (NIV)

² "So when you give to the needy, do not announce it with trumpets, as the hypocrites do in the

synagogues and on the streets, to be honored by others. Truly I tell you, they have received their reward in full.**

⁵ "And when you pray, do not be like the hypocrites, for they love to pray standing in the synagogues and on the street corners to be seen by others. Truly I tell you, they have received their reward in full.

¹⁶ "When you fast, do not look somber as the hypocrites do, for they disfigure their faces to show others they are fasting. Truly I tell you, they have received their reward in full.

Giving is a topic that can put people on the defense. I have a lot of friends that are newer Christians and aren't fully submitted to God in this area, and they get a little uncomfortable with it. I always go back to Matthew 6, which talks about praying, giving, and fasting. I feel like these three things are a cord of three strands that can't be easily broken. If you can get these three areas of your life dialed in and submit to the Lord, it will be life changing. If you are only doing one piece or two pieces, you are missing out on the power of all three.

There's a Bible story that I love in 1 Kings 17 (NIV), about a single mom who had a little boy. She was a widow and really struggling during a famine. She was broke, and the food was scarce. All that she had was a handful of flour in one jar and some olive oil, exactly enough ingredients to make one meal, which

I am assuming was bread. So, she decided that she and her son were going to eat one last meal, and then they would both die because they had no more food. She figured they would only live as long as that last meal would sustain them. Elijah was affected by this same famine, and God told him that he wanted him to go to a certain town and find the widow who would supply him with food. It is so bizarre that God was asking him to do that because widows were already struggling, especially during a famine! So, he goes and meets the widow I just mentioned, who tells him that it was her last meal that she had left. And this is crazy, but Elijah told the widow that he wanted her to give him the last of the bread, and after he ate some, they could have the rest for themselves. And then he said "PS, if you do it in this order where you feed me first and then feed yourselves, you will never run out of flour and oil until the famine ends and God sends rain." The widow did it, she gave the bread to Elijah first, and then she went back and the ingredients were replenished. This kept happening over and over again. Her flour and oil never ran dry as every day she had just enough ingredients to make the bread. It would have been really easy for this lady to deny Elijah's request and tell him that he was crazy! But she had faith and generosity, and because of that, God continuously re-supplied her jars.

I love the story of the widow because anytime God has called me to give way beyond what I think is normal, and when he really moves me to give so generously that I am scratching my head thinking "Oh my, what if I need this money later, what if God doesn't re-supply and I have an emergency?" I remember God's promises and the way that He provided for this widow because of her generosity and obedience.

Let's look at two people, Tim the Tither and Kim the Keeper. Tim decides he wants to live on 90% of his income and Kim decides she wants to live on 100% of her income and not tithe. But here's what happens to Kim. The dishwasher breaks, her car needs repair, she never has enough money and there is always something. Always an "emergency" that costs more money than she has.

I used to have a Black Range Rover and I had this friend who said "Beware! I have a Range Rover and every time I turn around, my Range Rover needs something-a new transmission, brakes, or headlights." I drove that car for years and hardly ever had issues! I felt like this was God's provision. Tim the Tither knew that he would rather live on 90% of his income with God's blessing than 100% of his income without God's blessing. Kim thinks that she is going to be better off with 100% of her money, but she is walking in disobedience with God and is missing out on his blessings. If Kim and Tim both have financial goals, such as having a set amount they know they want to put in their savings, I can guarantee you Tim is going to have a better time reaching that goal with 90% of his income than Kim is with 100% of her income. I can't explain it, but I've seen it over and over again. I have a friend who always gave really sporadically. Sometimes she would tithe, sometimes she wouldn't, depending on the month that she had extra. She decided that she wanted to set up an auto draft to come out of her paycheck twice a week. She knew she needed to be consistent and stop making excuses, and felt the auto draft was the best way to keep her commitment.

Not long after she set up the auto draft, she began seeing unexpected blessings in her life. First of all, her Grandpa called her out of the blue and said he wanted to bless her with money to put towards a down payment when she decided it was the time to buy her first house! Second, an owner of a gym who knew she had big fitness goals offered two months of free personal training. And finally, God provided a way for her to make more money at work by getting her real estate license. As soon as she did this, she started seeing real estate referrals come in. When my friend set up her auto draft, she did it with the intentions of obedience and with a lot of faith. She didn't do it because she thought that if she gave, someone would call and offer her a down payment! God honored her faith and obedience in ways she could have never seen coming. She recently told me that when she receives a commission check or a gift or something that is unexpected, she actually feels excited to give an extra tithe. She now sees these unexpected blessings as an opportunity to give God even more.

I am so glad God blessed my friend in this way, but I want to be clear that sometimes when you give, you're not going to see an immediate fruit, or an immediate check showing up in your mailbox. But it is crazy to see how many friends I've seen that as soon as they step out in faith with their first tithe, they receive an immediate blessing.

The only place in the whole Bible where God says "test me" is in reference to tithing:

Malachi 3:10 (NIV) Bring the whole tithe into the storehouse, that there may be food in my house.

Test me in this," says the LORD Almighty, "and see if I will not throw open the floodgates of heaven and pour out so much blessing that there will not be room enough to store it.

In every other place in the Bible, you'll see that we shouldn't test God or put Him to the test. But when it comes to tithing, not only does He say that it's okay to test God, but it's actually encouraged. And I see story after story of people who see a reward on their first tithe when they test God. It happened to me. When I felt led to start tithing, I was making $300 per week. I wrote a check for $30 knowing I didn't have $30 in my account! But the whole sermon at church was about testing and tithing, so I wrote the check. The next day, when I checked my mail, I got a check from Dominion Power that was for a $300 deposit that I paid seven years ago! It was a mistake on their end that took so long, that they even gave me some interest. Talk about providing! It's the hardest to get started on tithing when you are like I was, or like my friend, or the widow in the Bible, but the Bible makes it clear that we are called to tithe no matter how much or little money we have:

Luke 16:10 (NIV) Whoever can be trusted with very little can also be trusted with much, and whoever is dishonest with very little will also be dishonest with much.

You can't look for God to reward you in your finances without giving and praying in addition to your fasting. I love the following verse:

Joel 2:15, 18-19, 24-25 NIV

[15] Blow the trumpet in Zion,

declare a holy fast,

call a sacred assembly.

[18] Then the Lord was jealous for his land

and took pity on his people.

[19] The Lord replied to them:

"I am sending you grain, new wine and olive oil,

enough to satisfy you fully;

never again will I make you

an object of scorn to the nations.

[24] The threshing floors will be filled with grain;

the vats will overflow with new wine and oil.

[25] "I will repay you for the years the locusts have eaten—

the great locust and the young locust,

the other locusts and the locust swarm—

my great army that I sent among you.

A locust invasion represents poverty. The locusts came and devoured Israel's harvest. Joel gathered the people to fast and God rewarded them with grain, wine, and oil, all of which represents prosperity. I believe that fasting, giving, and praying breaks this spirit of financial struggle.

One time I took my son, Kyle, to McDonald's to get him some french fries. I didn't want any so I didn't order for myself. They smelled good though, so as he was eating his, I reached to grab one.

Kyle said, "You can't have any; these are MY fries!"

I had three thoughts.

First of all, Kyle forgot that I was the source of all fries. He wouldn't have any fries if it weren't for me. I drove him to McDonald's, ordered, and paid for the fries. Without me, there are no fries.

Second, Kyle didn't realize that I could take all of those fries away in an instant if I wanted. I could also go back and buy him a truckload of fries if I wanted to. I was totally in charge of the amount of fries he had or didn't have.

Third, I didn't need his fries. I could have bought my own fries if I wanted to. I could go back through the drive-thru and get my own. What I wanted him to learn was unselfishness. I wanted him to learn to share.

God does the same with us. He doesn't need our money. The money He has given us is all His. He just loaned it to us. Everything we have now is from God, directly. He can take away everything or give you ten times the amount instantly. God is the giver of all fries, and He is generous!

Proverbs 21:26 (NLT)

26 Some people are always greedy for more,

but the godly love to give!

We're all familiar with John 3:16:

John 3:16 (NIV)

¹⁶ For God so loved the world that he gave his one and only Son, that whoever believes in him shall not perish but have eternal life.

You can give without loving, but you can't love without giving. Generosity is important. You should really try to give each year a little more than you did the year before. I hear people say if they made more money they would be happy to give, but the truth is you wouldn't. I gave when I made $9/hour while working 20 hours a week.

Proverbs 14:31 (NIV)

³¹ Whoever oppresses the poor shows contempt for their Maker, but whoever is kind to the needy honors God.

Matthew 6:21 (NIV)

²¹ For where your treasure is, there your heart will be also.

I lived on $9/hour working 20 hours a week struggling to pay bills and putting things on credit cards. I was in a bad place financially, but God told me He needed me to trust Him and give Him 10%. It wasn't a lot of money, but for me it was an enormous amount. God kept encouraging me to tithe. If you think you can't give anything because you don't have enough, I want to encourage you to just trust him.

2 Corinthians 9:13 (NIV)

13 Because of the service by which you have proved yourselves, others will praise God for the obedience that accompanies your confession of the gospel of Christ, and for your generosity in sharing with them and with everyone else.

Your giving proves the reality of your faith.

Philemon 1:6 (NIV)

6 I pray that your partnership with us in the faith may be effective in deepening your understanding of every good thing we share for the sake of Christ.

You are generous because of your faith.

Malachi 3:10 (NIV)

10 Bring the whole tithe into the storehouse, that there may be food in my house. Test me in this," says the Lord Almighty, "and see if I will not throw open the floodgates of heaven and pour out so much blessing that there will not be room enough to store it.

God dares you to trust His promises!

When I tell you to give, you know I don't have a dog in this race. I'm not asking you to give to me. Whether or not you give is up to you, but you are missing out on God's blessings on your life by not doing it.

Fasting is going to help increase your faith, but you also need to be willing to give. This is a hard area for people to breakthrough in, but it's very important. I used to work for a church where a pastor on staff was fired because he wasn't tithing.

Here are some scriptures for financial breakthrough you can paraphrase in your own words:

- **Psalm 1:3 (NIV) I yield fruit in season. My leaves do not wither and whatever I do prospers.**
- **Joel 2:24 (NIV) My threshing floors will be filled with grain and overflow with oil.**
- **Proverbs 3:10 (NIV) My barns are filled to overflowing and my vats brim over with new wine**

PART 2: FASTING FOR PROTECTION

The book of Ezra tells the story of Jews traveling back from captivity in Persia. Ezra was a priest and he basically led a second group of people back to Jerusalem. Ezra really needed protection while he led them across the wilderness to the Promised Land.

Ezra 8:22-23 (NIV)

22 I was ashamed to ask the king for soldiers and horsemen to protect us from enemies on the road, because we had told the king, "The gracious hand of our God is on everyone who looks to him, but his great anger is against all who forsake him." **23** So we fasted and petitioned our God about this, and he answered our prayer.

Here are some other verses that talk about that hedge of protection:

Job 1:10-12 (NIV)

10 "Have you not put a hedge around him and his household and everything he has? You have blessed the work of his hands, so that his flocks and herds are spread throughout the land. **11** But now stretch out your hand and strike everything he has, and he will surely curse you to your face."

12 The LORD said to Satan, "Very well, then, everything he has is in your power, but on the man himself do not lay a finger."

Then Satan went out from the presence of the LORD.

Luke 22:31-32 (NIV)

³¹ "Simon, Simon, Satan has asked to sift all of you as wheat. ³² But I have prayed for you, Simon, that your faith may not fail. And when you have turned back, strengthen your brothers."

Here are three things we can gather from these passages:

- As followers of Christ, we have a hedge of protection placed around us by God.
- Satan must get permission to do anything inside that hedge.
- Even when Satan has permission, God places restrictions on what he does.

Esther 4:15-16 (NIV)

Then Esther sent this reply to Mordecai: "Go, gather together all the Jews who are in Susa, and fast for me. Do not eat or drink for three days, night or day. I and my attendants will fast as you do. When this is done, I will go to the king, even though it is against the law. And if I perish, I perish."

Esther 5:9-13 (NIV)

⁹ Haman went out that day happy and in high spirits. But when he saw Mordecai at the king's gate and observed that he neither rose nor showed fear in his presence, he was filled with rage against Mordecai.

10 Nevertheless, Haman restrained himself and went home.

Calling together his friends and Zeresh, his wife, **11** Haman boasted to them about his vast wealth, his many sons, and all the ways the king had honored him and how he had elevated him above the other nobles and officials. **12** "And that's not all," Haman added. "I'm the only person Queen Esther invited to accompany the king to the banquet she gave. And she has invited me along with the king tomorrow. **13** But all this gives me no satisfaction as long as I see that Jew Mordecai sitting at the king's gate."

Everything looked like it was going according to Haman's plan, but Esther had prayed and fasted for her meeting with the king. She knew she could be killed for approaching the king without being summoned, so she called a corporate fast involving all of her people. This is a perfect example of the power of getting a bunch of believers together to fast and pray about the same thing at the same time.

Esther 7:2-6 (NIV)

2 and as they were drinking wine on the second day, the king again asked, "Queen Esther, what is your petition? It will be given you. What is your request? Even up to half the kingdom, it will be granted."

³ Then Queen Esther answered, "If I have found favor with you, Your Majesty, and if it pleases you, grant me my life—this is my petition. And spare my people—this is my request. ⁴ For I and my people have been sold to be destroyed, killed and annihilated. If we had merely been sold as male and female slaves, I would have kept quiet, because no such distress would justify disturbing the king."

⁵ King Xerxes asked Queen Esther, "Who is he? Where is he—the man who has dared to do such a thing?"

⁶ Esther said, "An adversary and enemy! This vile Haman!"

Then Haman was terrified before the king and queen.

This story ends with the death of Haman, which meant protection for all of the Jews.

SPIRITUAL WARFARE

When it comes to protection, there is no better protection than the armor of God. The Bible says to put on the full armor of God and not to be a slave to the Devil. I've been asked before, "Chantel, you don't really believe in the Devil, do you?" I respond with, "Absolutely, I do!"

There are a lot of people, believe it or not, that don't believe in the Devil. They are well meaning Christians that believe in God, but they don't believe in the Devil. If you are going to defeat your enemy, you need to understand how the enemy works. The Devil is not a superstition. He's not a figment of the imagination and he's not a character with a pitchfork. The Devil is very real. He is a liar, a thief, and a killer, and he's out to destroy your life. He hates every person that loves, serves, and worships God.

The Devil and his demons are real. They try to get you to stumble and doubt God. The Devil is really deceptive and very strategic. He takes his time and he makes you think you're winning. You can be doing the wrong things and he'll deceive you into thinking that those things are okay. He's constantly putting ideas into your mind attacking your marriage, your home, and your family. The fights you have with your spouse aren't a coincidence. It's playing right into the Devil's hands. The Devil wants you to be angry and divided. He wants you defeated and out of his way. You need to recognize when the Devil is at work and tell him, "Look! I'm no fool. I'm not going to fall for your shenanigans. No!"

The Devil tempts with thoughts in the mind. If I'm eating and I'm already full, I can hear him telling me, "Just take one more bite. It's so good. There are only three bites left. You might as well finish it." When he's trying to attack my marriage he'll say, "Your husband is always getting angry about stupid stuff. He doesn't really care about you."

Here's an example. At the time that I'm writing this, Easter just passed and I like to give things away. I was having a conversation with a woman and asked her how her Easter was. She said that money was tight and she didn't do anything for her children. I decided to give her our leftover Easter candy which happened to include a pack of Cadbury Eggs my kids' grandfather bought for them. Later that afternoon, my husband came home and asked what happened to the Cadbury eggs. I told him. He said, "Those weren't yours to give away. You should have asked the kids before you did that." I told him that I could just buy more if it was that important to him. Before you knew it, we were in a blowout argument over $1.99 Cadbury eggs! I thought, "This is the Devil! This is insanity that we're fighting over this right now."

You have to notice these kinds of things. Look out for the Devil's tactics and use the Word of God to put a stop to it. Don't let the Devil in. I've seen Christians visiting psychics for fun, listening to the things they tell them and getting excited when they get something right about their lives. Of course they got it right. It's spiritual wickedness and you just allowed the Devil into your life. Don't play those games with the Devil.

Ephesians 6:12 (NIV)

[12] For our struggle is not against flesh and blood, but against the rulers, against the authorities, against the powers of this dark world and against the spiritual forces of evil in the heavenly realms.

If you try to fight the devil in your own power, you're not going to win. You can only win with spiritual weapons.

2 Corinthians 10:4 (NIV)

⁴ The weapons we fight with are not the weapons of the world. On the contrary, they have divine power to demolish strongholds.

Mark 9:29 (NKJV)

²⁹ So He said to them, "This kind can come out by nothing but prayer and fasting."

See that last scripture? Mark 9:29 is the key to this whole book. Let's look into this chapter a little more.

Mark 9:14-19, 25-29 (NKJV)

¹⁴ And when He came to the disciples, He saw a great multitude around them, and scribes disputing with them. ¹⁵ Immediately, when they saw Him, all the people were greatly amazed, and running to *Him,* greeted Him. ¹⁶ And He asked the scribes, "What are you discussing with them?"

¹⁷ Then one of the crowd answered and said, "Teacher, I brought You my son, who has a mute spirit. ¹⁸ And wherever it seizes him, it throws him

down; he foams at the mouth, gnashes his teeth, and becomes rigid. So I spoke to Your disciples, that they should cast it out, but they could not."

[19] He answered him and said, "O faithless generation, how long shall I be with you? How long shall I bear with you? Bring him to Me."

[25] When Jesus saw that the people came running together, He rebuked the unclean spirit, saying to it: "Deaf and dumb spirit, I command you, come out of him and enter him no more!" [26] Then *the spirit* cried out, convulsed him greatly, and came out of him. And he became as one dead, so that many said, "He is dead." [27] But Jesus took him by the hand and lifted him up, and he arose.

[28] And when He had come into the house, His disciples asked Him privately, "Why could we not cast it out?"

[29] So He said to them, "This kind can come out by nothing but prayer and fasting."

This is the way we have to fight. You may say, "Well, I don't have a demonic power inside of me." Well, I think that if you have a struggle you can't beat that overtakes you over and over and over again, then that's exactly what it is. It's not just a physical problem. It's a spiritual force.

FIGHTING TEMPTATION

Almost everyone has their personal temptations they fight with every day. It can be a temptation to abuse food, alcohol, pornography, or drugs. It can be a temptation to have sex outside of marriage, gossip, or overspend. If we're honest, most of us will admit that we're losing our fight with temptation more than we're winning.

In Matthew 4. the Devil tried to tempt Jesus:

Matthew 4:2-3 (NIV)

[2] After fasting forty days and forty nights, he was hungry. [3] The tempter came to him and said, "If you are the Son of God, tell these stones to become bread."

It's ironic that food was the first temptation he challenged Jesus with. It's also the temptation Satan got Adam and Eve with. He still uses food today. There's nothing wrong with food, but like with all material things, Satan tempts you to use food out of the boundaries God has set for us.

Matthew 4:4 (NIV)

[4] Jesus answered, "It is written: 'Man shall not live on bread alone, but on every word that comes from the mouth of God."

Jesus combated Satan's temptation with "it is written."

Matthew 4:5 (NIV)

⁵ Then the devil took him to the holy city and had him stand on the highest point of the temple.

Did you know that Satan knows the Bible and will even quote it to you? He quotes it correctly but applies it incorrectly. He distorts its application. There's a funny story I heard once about a man who believed God wanted him to have an affair with another's man wife. His defense was Philippians 4:13 (NKJV) "I can do all things through Christ who strengthens me."

Matthew 4:6-11 (NIV)

⁶ "If you are the Son of God," he said, "throw yourself down. For it is written:

"He will command his angels concerning you, and they will lift you up in their hands, so that you will not strike your foot against a stone."

⁷ Jesus answered him, "It is also written: 'Do not put the Lord your God to the test.'"

⁸ Again, the devil took him to a very high mountain and showed him all the kingdoms of the world and their splendor. ⁹ "All this I will give you," he said, "if you will bow down and worship me."

10 Jesus said to him, "Away from me, Satan! For it is written: 'Worship the Lord your God, and serve him only.'"

11 Then the devil left him, and angels came and attended him.

Jesus countered Satan with "it is written" in the last two temptations just like He did in the first. The temptation may not leave immediately when you first quote a scripture, but that doesn't mean you stop. Sometimes you have to quote the Word multiple times.

James 4:7 (NIV)

7 Submit yourselves, then, to God. Resist the devil, and he will flee from you.

The Word promises us that if we resist the Devil's temptation, he will flee from us. How did Jesus resist the Devil? He used the Word. He threw Scripture in the Devil's face like snowballs. Fighting with our own willpower and determination won't win the battle.

You can tell yourself, "I won't gossip today" as much as you like, but if you keep blowing it over and over again you'll realize that doesn't work on its own. Jesus just showed us what weapons we're supposed to use.

Ephesians 6:11, 17 (NIV)

11 Put on the full armor of God, so that you can take your stand against the devil's schemes.

17 Take the helmet of salvation and the sword of the Spirit, which is the word of God.

Our #1 weapon is the Word of God!

Hebrews 4:12 (NIV)

12 For the word of God is alive and active. Sharper than any double-edged sword, it penetrates even to dividing soul and spirit, joints and marrow; it judges the thoughts and attitudes of the heart.

2 Corinthians 10:3-4 (NIV)

3 For though we live in the world, we do not wage war as the world does.4 The weapons we fight with are not the weapons of the world. On the contrary, they have divine power to demolish strongholds.

The weapons of the world are willpower, grit and determination. The weapons of the Christian believer have divine power! This is why we have to memorize Scripture. It's our divine weapon. If you only learn one thing from this book, I want you to learn this. This principle is something I'm going to talk about over and over again because hearing it once is not enough.

Find scriptures that deal with your recurring temptation. If you struggle with resisting the urge to have premarital sex or an addiction to pornography, then 1 Thessalonians 4:3 is for you.

1 Thessalonians 4:3 (NIV)

3 It is God's will that you should be sanctified: that you should avoid sexual immorality;

If you struggle with being a gossiper, quote Ephesians 4:29:

Ephesians 4:29 (NIV)

29 Do not let any unwholesome talk come out of your mouths, but only what is helpful for building others up according to their needs, that it may benefit those who listen.

If you're someone who cuts corners and battles with laziness, you can use Colossians 3:23:

Colossians 3:23 (NIV)

23 Whatever you do, work at it with all your heart, as working for the Lord, not for human masters,

Do you struggle with anxiety?

Philippians 4:6 (NIV)

6 Do not be anxious about anything, but in every situation, by prayer and petition, with thanksgiving, present your requests to God.

How about fear?

Isaiah 43:2-4 (NIV)

2 When you pass through the waters,

I will be with you;

and when you pass through the rivers,

they will not sweep over you.

When you walk through the fire,

you will not be burned;

the flames will not set you ablaze.

3 For I am the Lord your God,

the Holy One of Israel, your Savior;

I give Egypt for your ransom,

Cush and Seba in your stead.

4 Since you are precious and honored in my sight,

and because I love you,

I will give people in exchange for you,

nations in exchange for your life.

Before you make that wrong decision, attack the Devil with the Word.

"It is written …"

"It is written …"

"It is written …"

It may sound easy, but it's not easy when you're being tempted and you feel weak. However, it's what Jesus did to fight Satan and it worked. You have two options. Keep doing it your way that doesn't work, or do it Jesus' way.

Psalm 119:11 (NIV)

11 I have hidden your word in my heart that I might not sin against you.

Jesus had Scripture available to use against Satan because he had been meditating on the book of Deuteronomy where he got those verses from. I meditate in the Word and write Bible verses down on index cards. On the other side of the card, I write the problem it's associated with (i.e. anger, fear, overeating)

If you want to change your Christian walk, memorizing Scripture and putting it in your heart will do it tenfold.

THE ARMOR OF GOD

In Ephesians 6, the apostle Paul talks about the "full armor of God" we need to put on.

Ephesians 6:13 (NIV)

13 Therefore put on the full armor of God, so that when the day of evil comes, you may be able to stand

---

your ground, and after you have done everything,

to stand.

I want to point out "when the day of evil comes." Paul said *when*, not if. That means we already know that evil is going to come our way.

Ephesians 6:14a (NIV)

¹⁴ Stand firm then, with the belt of truth buckled

around your waist …

People often lie to themselves, and as a result they defeat themselves. They don't do it on purpose. You need to put on the belt of truth. What is the belt of truth? It's integrity. It's not lying to yourself. What is the breastplate of righteousness? It's purity. Guard your heart. Hold yourself accountable for who you hang out with, what you watch, and what you listen to. Guard your heart with that breastplate of purity.

Whatever issue you struggle with is the one you need to focus on. I give a lot of examples about food and overeating because that was always my struggle. So, using me as an example, I have to be careful who I spend a lot of time with because I have a few friends that like to eat, eat, eat! I have to be careful not to get caught up when I go out with them. It's important to recognize what stage of resistance you're at because there may be some people you have to distance yourself from for a season. Eventually, though, you may get to a place where being around the temptation doesn't bother you at all.

I used to smoke, but when I was 22-years-old, I decided to quit. In the beginning, I couldn't hang out with a lot of the people I used to because they still smoked. I knew that if I did, I would be right back where I started.

Ephesians 6:14b (NIV)

14 ··· with the breastplate of righteousness in place,

According to Ephesians 6:14 (AMPC), it is the "breastplate of integrity." You need integrity, or honesty, to break free from bondage in your life. You have to be honest about it.

I always saw integrity as a core trait of mine, but before I lost weight I wasn't honest about my relationship with food. I told myself all kinds of lies:

"The reason I'm overweight isn't because of overeating. It's because of my thyroid problems. I'm overweight because my husband is stressing me out and I run a business with over 200 employees."

It wasn't intentional, but I was letting Satan feed me these lies over and over again to keep me in bondage.

The other day I came home from a long day at work feeling like I needed a pick-me-up. I decided to eat some gummy bears. I wasn't hungry and I could feel God telling me I shouldn't eat them. As soon as I started chewing, the crown of my tooth came out! I had no business eating those gummy bears in the first place.

Ephesians 6:15 (NIV)

15 and with your feet fitted with the readiness that comes from the gospel of peace.

Peace doesn't mean you don't have storms. It means you have peace despite the storms.

Mark 4:35-40 (NIV)

35 That day when evening came, he said to his disciples, "Let us go over to the other side." 36 Leaving the crowd behind, they took him along, just as he was, in the boat. There were also other boats with him. 37 A furious squall came up, and the waves broke over the boat, so that it was nearly swamped. 38 Jesus was in the stern, sleeping on a cushion. The disciples woke him and said to him, "Teacher, don't you care if we drown?"

39 He got up, rebuked the wind and said to the waves, "Quiet! Be still!" Then the wind died down and it was completely calm.

40 He said to his disciples, "Why are you so afraid? Do you still have no faith?"

As a Christian, you can decide to have peace when you see the Devil attacking you. If you have a bad report from your doctor, your kids are falling away, or you have trouble in your friendships, you can still have God's peace in your life.

Ephesians 6:16 (NIV)

[16] In addition to all this, take up the shield of faith, with which you can extinguish all the flaming arrows of the evil one.

Paul was imprisoned in Rome when he wrote this. I can imagine him looking at the armor and the shields of the Roman soldiers keeping him locked up and using what the Devil had done to him against him. You can imagine the kind of faith Paul had when he wrote this. This blows my mind, because I think I have a lot of faith, but if I ended up in a jail cell by the will of God, I don't know where my faith would be.

In a situation like that, my mind would be challenged with doubts like "where is God?" That's what Satan does all the time. He always seeds doubt in your mind. I hear doubt all the time from the listeners of my *"Waist Away"* podcast who write me questions. They'll experience some weight loss with intermittent fasting, but when they gain a pound or two they question if they should keep going. That's the Devil at work trying to make you doubt where you are and what you're doing.

He speaks into your mind thoughts of defeat like, "God's never going to free you from overeating. God's never going to prosper you. You're a failure. You're never going to fulfill your dreams."

When the Devil starts talking you have to put up the shield of faith. Say, "This is what God told me. He is my healer. He is my success. He is my victory. He is going to deliver me from this."

That's what I had to do. I had to tell the Devil that I refused to be in bondage anymore. I had to decide to be free from over- and emotional eating. I had to say these things and quote God's promises in His Word at the same time.

Create a series of positive statements about yourself that you can confess every day. Here are mine that I say every morning:

1. I develop leaders. It's not something I do; it's who I am.

2. I give my very best and then some every single day.

3. God, show me how I can be a blessing in someone else's life today.

4. God, show me how I can grow closer to you, and how I can help others grow closer to you.

5. I will eat food for fuel and not for any other reason.

When I go for a walk, I speak to God. I say, "God, I am going to put on the breastplate of righteousness. Lord don't lead me into temptation. Help me to not focus on food. Help me to focus on Your Word this morning. Protect my body from my head to my toes. Help me to have faith that you're going to keep healing my body. Help me to eat clean, healthy food. Please keep the Devil away from me today. I don't want to be a slave to food anymore. I want to praise you for healing my body from my head to my toes. Thank you for healing any psoriasis in my body, Father. Keep my thyroid functioning at the highest capacity. I want to wear the whole armor of God this morning. I want to have shoes of peace. I want to have the shield of faith and I want to have victory in my life over this bondage of eating today."

That's a powerful prayer. "Suit up" in prayer every single morning. Another huge component to this is memorizing Scripture! When Satan came to Jesus with "If you are the Son of God," Jesus came back with His Sword (the Word).

"It is written!" *Chop!*

"It is written!" *Slice!*

"It is written!" *Stab!*

Then what happened? Satan left!

FLEEING TEMPTATION

Temptation is the desire to do something wrong that you know you will regret in the morning. My greatest temptation in life is overeating. I lived in a home that encouraged using food to deal with pain, pleasure, and every other emotion. Whether it's drugs, sex, pornography, or something else, everyone has some sort of temptation they deal with and a lot of us lose the battle more than we win. As followers of Jesus Christ, God gave us weapons that we can use to win the battle.

Matthew 4:1 (NIV)

Then Jesus was led by the Spirit into the wilderness to be tempted by the devil.

Why was the Devil tempting the Lord Jesus to sin? Because if Satan could get Jesus to commit even one sin, he could get rid of God's plan of salvation forever.

God's plan was **substitutionary atonement**, using a substitute to atone for your sin and my sin. However, the substitute had to be sinless and without blemish because God's justice cannot let someone pay our death penalty when they owe a death penalty themselves.

1 Peter 1:18-19 (NIV)

18 For you know that it was not with perishable things such as silver or gold that you were redeemed from the empty way of life handed down to you from your ancestors, 19 but with the precious blood of Christ, a lamb without blemish or defect.

It says a lamb without blemish or defect. Underline that important phrase. There would have been huge consequence if Satan had gotten Jesus to sin on even one thing.

Matthew 4:2-3 (NIV)

2 After fasting forty days and forty nights, he was hungry. 3 The tempter came to him and said, "If you are the Son of God, tell these stones to become bread."

The first temptation was food. The first temptation in the Garden of Eden was food, too. It was God's will that Jesus go without food at this moment in His life, so Satan was trying to have Jesus do his own will for His life.

Matthew 4:4 (NIV)

4 Jesus answered, "It is written: 'Man shall not live on bread alone, but on every word that comes from the mouth of God.'

Jesus said it was better to be hungry in the will of God than to be satisfied outside of the will of God. Jesus had now gone 40 days without food and water. When I miss one day of eating, I'm willing to eat my arm off!

Matthew 4:5-7 (NIV)

5 Then the devil took him to the holy city and had him stand on the highest point of the temple. 6 "If you are the Son of God," he said, "throw yourself down. For it is written:

"'He will command his angels concerning you, and they will lift you up in their hands, so that you will not strike your foot against a stone.'"

7 Jesus answered him, "It is also written: 'Do not put the Lord your God to the test.'"

Isn't it amazing that Satan is quoting the Bible? He takes God's Word and twists it. First he tempts with food. Second, he tempts with pride. We're tempted in these two areas all the time.

Matthew 4:8-9 (NIV)

8 Again, the devil took him to a very high mountain

and showed him all the kingdoms of the world and

their splendor. 9 "All this I will give you," he said,

"if you will bow down and worship me."

Satan was trying to offer a way for Jesus to avoid the hardship and pain of dying on the cross. He tried to use what was promised Jesus in Psalm 2:

Psalm 2:7-8 (NIV)

7 I will proclaim the Lord's decree:

He said to me, "You are my son;

today I have become your father.

8 Ask me,

and I will make the nations your inheritance,

the ends of the earth your possession.

The Devil was trying to tempt Jesus to think he could skip the plan of salvation and still be on the throne. But for Jesus, God's way to the throne was by the cross.

Matthew 4:10 (NIV)

[10] Jesus said to him, "Away from me, Satan! For it is written: 'Worship the Lord your God, and serve him only.'"

James 4:7 (NIV)

[7] Submit yourselves, then, to God. Resist the devil, and he will flee from you.

Chapter 16

FASTING TO BREAK THE BONDAGE OF AN ENSLAVING SIN

In my opinion, the #1 reason to fast is to be freed from the bondage of sin. The sins that bind you in a way that you feel like a victim to them are what I call enslaving sins. These aren't "heat of the moment" sins that you don't do often. If a friend asks you how their new outfit looks and you lie and tell them it looks great then, yes, that is a sin, but it isn't an enslaving sin. Enslaving sins are those problems that are a recurring theme over and over in your life. They're the sins that you tried everything to free yourself from but couldn't.

The best analogy that I can think of for enslaving sins is this movie called "Groundhog Day" where a guy was forced to live the same day over and over again, the whole movie repeats that one day! Kind of like the movie "50 First Dates" In which Drew Barrymore had a memory problem, so every date with Adam Sandler was like a first date. Every day you wake up and your same ole' sin is on repeat.

Maybe your enslaving sin is overspending: you wake up, and the next thing you know, you are walking into a store and buying things you don't need.

Maybe your enslaving sin is porn, and you say "I am never watching it again," and then you continue to repeat the pattern every day. Maybe your enslaving sin is overeating and you say, "I am never going to binge again," but the cycle repeats.

Even if you love God, you can still live a defeated life when you are constantly living Groundhog Day with your enslaving sin. This type of Groundhog Day can keep you from seeing a breakthrough if you don't stop the repetitive cycle!

I have a lot of friends that are single and are really searching for a godly mate. I believe that one of the reasons people aren't able to find a mate is because of their enslaving sins.

I have a single friend who is about 100-150 pounds overweight and has an enslaving sin to food. She is upset that she hasn't found a husband and really wants to get married. One of the reasons why she might not be finding a husband is because she is struggling with this enslaving sin. She has to get to a point where she says "I want this husband more than I want to be a slave to food." This particular issue may be blocking her from the reward of a husband. Maybe your enslaving sin is pornography and you seek a godly spouse. You have to conquer this sin before you can have a godly because you are setting your marriage up for major issues if you go into it with a pornography addiction. If your enslaving sin is overspending and you are going into debt to do so, how can you expect to attract a godly, responsible, secure spouse when you can't get your own affairs in order?

Ask yourself, does the reward outweigh the sacrifice? Your enslaving sin can't be broken with ordinary willpower. You are fasting so that you can release that bondage of sin.

Matthew 17:14-20 (NIV)

[14] When they came to the crowd, a man approached Jesus and knelt before him. [15] "Lord, have mercy on my son," he said. "He has seizures and is suffering greatly. He often falls into the fire or into the water. [16] I brought him to your disciples, but they could not heal him."

[17] "You unbelieving and perverse generation," Jesus replied, "how long shall I stay with you? How long shall I put up with you? Bring the boy here to me." [18] Jesus rebuked the demon, and it came out of the boy, and he was healed at that moment.

[19] Then the disciples came to Jesus in private and asked, "Why couldn't we drive it out?"

[20] He replied, "Because you have so little faith. Truly I tell you, if you have faith as small as a mustard seed, you can say to this mountain, 'Move from here to there,' and it will move. Nothing will be impossible for you."

The demon in these verses is an example of an enslaving sin. The most common enslaving sins I've seen Christians in bondage to are compulsive overeating, alcohol, drugs, pornography, and tobacco. But there are so many others, such as gossip, anxiety/lack of trusting God, dishonesty, overspending and poor money management. Just to name a few!

Use the following statements to identify if the problem you're dealing with is an enslaving sin.

1. I've tried over and over and I can't break the cycle.

2. I don't want to do this, but I can't seem to help myself. I keep getting stuck in the same rut over and over.

3. I need to break free, but I can't seem to find the way.

If these three statements are true for your situation, then you know you're dealing with an enslaving sin.

Let's look at Matthew 17:1-26 (NIV) again. The boy's father didn't understand what was wrong with the boy. Jesus knew that a demon had entered into the boy and taken control of his life. Today, we hesitate to identify a problem as demon possession because it sounds spooky. At the same time, if we have one of these enslaving sins, this means that we've allowed Satan to come into this part of our lives and keep lying to us over and over about the issue. For example, my enslaving sin was overeating, and I believed little lies that encouraged me to eat more than I had to. If I felt sick, I would eat more. If the food tasted really good, I would make it my only meal of the day so I could overeat. Whenever I was stressed, I believed I needed junk food for comfort.

An enslaving sin is any sin that can't be broken with ordinary willpower.

It's exactly how it sounds. You're enslaved to it. Jesus told his disciples:

Matthew 17:20 (NIV)

"...Truly I tell you, if you have faith as small as a mustard seed, you can say to this mountain, 'Move from here to there,' and it will move. Nothing will be impossible for you."

STEPS FOR DEFEATING AN ENSLAVING SIN

#1 List the Lies

Write out the lies you believe that keep you bound. The enslaving sin I dealt with was overeating, so here are some of my examples: **I don't want to waste food.** It's the human trash can excuse. Excess food is going to be wasted one way or another. It's either going in the trash can or in your body. Do you really want your body to be the trash can?

- **I'm so tired.** If you aren't undernourished, eating food doesn't give you a sudden burst of energy. It makes you more tired. It may give you a sugar high for ten minutes, but that's it.

- **I'm so stressed out.** Food, drugs, and alcohol can temporarily ease your stress but after ten minutes you're going to be more stressed!

- **I hardly ever get to eat XYZ.** It's the fear of missing out, right? My Iranian family makes really good food, and they only come to town every couple of months. So, I think *I'm never going to get kebob this good again for a long time*! But that isn't true. I can always get it again.

- **This tastes so good.** Not a good excuse! Food tastes better the hungrier you are. Actually, if you practice fasting, you'll often eat food when you're hungrier and end up enjoying it more!

- **I'm on vacation.** This is an excuse for doing anything I want!

- **I have eaten so clean all day, so I need to reward myself.** Junk food is not a reward for clean eating.

- **I might get hungry later.** This is "preventative eating:" eating because you don't want to get hungry later.

List all of these things that you're saying to yourself. List as many as you possibly can. It's really important to share these in a group setting. We need to list all of these things so that we can recognize them. So, when the lies come up again, you can fight them with Scripture.

You should also list the lies that Satan tells you.

Lies Vs Truth

Lie: This is just too hard, it is not good for my body or my metabolism.

Truth: **Romans 5:3 (NIV)- Not only so, but we also glory in our sufferings because we know suffering produces perseverance, perseverance character, and character, hope.**

One time, I went to hear John Maxwell speak and he put his hands in the air in a diagonal motion. He said "life is UP … hill … all … the … way" He kept repeating himself over and over again. I don't know why, but for me this was such a powerful statement, because he was saying no matter what we do in life, if it's going to have a good result, it's going to be a lot of hard work. If you are someone who doesn't embrace hard work, then you are not going to get anywhere. This is an uphill battle! Everyone wants this quick fix, and if they don't get it right away, they give up.

At the time I am writing this, my real estate brokerage has seven locations across the country. One of the things people ask us all the time when they are selling their house is what they should renovate? They want to know "Should I paint, redo the kitchen, etc?" We are constantly advising people what improvements will get them the biggest ROI. When I think about renovations, we are constantly dealing with contractors and stuff like that. My son, when he was little, even when he was under 2, he memorized this verse:

Romans 12:2 (NIV) Do not conform to the pattern of this world, but be transformed by the renewing of your mind. Then you will be able to test and approve what God's will is—his good, pleasing and perfect will.

As he got older, he asked me, what does it mean to renew your mind? I explained it to him with the example of home renovations. One of the things we've seen over and over with renovations is that it always takes longer than you think it's going to be. When I was thinking of this renewing of the mind, I realized it is like renovation of the mind, just like home improvements. It takes longer than you think. For me, I had to get to the place where I literally only used food for physical fuel. I had to get to a point where there was never ever a time that I would go to food when I wasn't physically hungry and didn't hear my stomach growling. When I was younger, my mom would day, she would say, "Let's get frozen yogurt." We would go to TCBY. If you are reading this and don't know what TCBY is, you are younger than me lol. This was like the old version of Pinkberry or Sweet Frogs. If I came home after a bad day she would say let's go to the mall and get some yogurt. I had to retrain my brain to say "Okay, I am having a bad day. I now need to run to God, call a friend, take a bath, go for a walk, or do anything else but run to food!" One of my friends Kristin Cutthriel says, "you have to sit with unease to cure the disease."

I have found myself doing it with my son Kyle. One time he was playing basketball with a couple of friends and one of them accidentally elbowed him in his eye. I was like, "Oh honey come inside; let's get you a lollipop. Will that make you feel better?" And I thought to myself, "Here I am trying to be a loving mom just like my mom was," but what I learned was that eating would make me feel better, and sweets are the cure to all my problems. The truth is that sweets are the cause of so many problems.

Let's switch gears to alcohol because the same is true. A lot of people watched their parents, anytime they had an argument or a bad day, make themselves a drink or pour a glass of wine.

There are things that you will have trouble removing. Think of renovating a house and when you want to put tile on the house now, for example. If you want to put tile over laminate, you don't even have to remove the laminate. If you have tile, and want to put laminate, you have to first remove the tile. Removing the tile takes so much work and effort. This is the problem: every time you get the urge to eat outside of when you are physically hungry, you have to take off all your old thoughts and put on new thoughts. You have to take off the lies and put on the truth. You cannot put laminate over top of tiles. You have to first remove the lies. You have to be honest and face the lies to begin with. If you are telling yourself, "I am fasting all day" but meanwhile you are having coffee with cream and sugar, you are not technically fasting. If you are having smoothies and juices, you aren't technically fasting. If you are saying, "Oh I am not doing this or that," but you actually are, you cannot make headway until you first strip down the old tile to put on the new wood floor.

One of the things you can do to renew your mind is to make a habit of creating a list of affirmations that you are going to say every day. Here are the affirmations that I say to myself:

I only eat when I am physically hungry.

I will never eat one more bite than my body is calling for.

I will never overeat.

I will never use food when I am stressed, happy, sad, or mad.

I understand that I am in a spiritual battle against Satan and I will break free from my stronghold of food.

I will run to God and quote Bible verses when I am tempted.

I will never use the line "I might as well eat because …"

You need to write down what the lies are and replace them with the truth, to set you free from bondage.

I want to share some really specific prayers and statements to make for some of these different enslaving sins you may be struggling with. Really, the prayers are interchangeable and most of them will apply to many different sins. The best thing you can do when you are making a proclamation is to quote words directly from the Bible, so many of these prayers below are based on Isaiah 58.

Food: In the name of Jesus, I pray that I lose the bondage of this eating issue. I understand that this is an emotional, heart issue and through God's power, I will break free.

Pornography: I command that every scheme of the devil that is driving me to turn to pornography is gone. I want you to undo the heavy burdens of pornography and I want the blood of Christ to take me to the next level in this area. I don't want to have a repeat year of this enslaved sin of pornography. I want you to break every yoke. I want your light to break forth!

Gossip: I command that every slanderous statement that I make or people make about me is unfruitful. My mouth is a tool of praise and testimony and will no longer be used to bring dishonor. Instead of spreading gossip, I ask that my light shall break forth like the morning, for your glory. I command that every hater I have is benched.

Negative Attitude: I ask that every blessing God has for me be fruitful and that multiplication shall come to pass. I know that God is for me and not against me, and His plans are for my good. Through God's power, I will undo the chains that my negative attitude hold over me. God, without you, I am going to lose my temper and get angry; I need your strength to keep me calm.

Feel free to customize these and make them your own!

My friend Kristin gave me an example when we were going for a walk. We try to walk together at least 2-3x week. One day she said, "Let me give you a perfect example of falling off the wagon. Let's say I was walking from House A to House B, and I fell a couple steps backwards because I tripped on something. If my goal is to get to House B, I am not going to walk backwards all the way back to house A, just because I fell a few steps back. I'm going to dust my pants off and keep walking to House B. When people fall off the wagon, they say, 'I am going to go all the way backwards, eat everything but the kitchen sink!' But that's such a lie. Just keep walking!" Let me give you an example of someone who may overeat even though they don't have a weight problem. But before I do, I am going to give an example of myself with drinking.

At my husband's 38th birthday party, everyone told me how great I looked and how skinny I looked. I didn't want to eat anything that night, but I was drinking an orange crush. If you don't know what an orange crush is, you need to go to Watermans in Virginia Beach. I am friends with the owner's wife, and she told me they sell more vodka to that restaurant than any other restaurant in Virginia. It's because of these crushes! So, I was drinking an orange crush, with fresh squeezed orange juice; you just suck it down because it's so delicious! So I had two drinks, and usually I would have been fine but since my stomach was empty, it was way too much for me to drink. I am not a big drinker, I literally drink 3 times a year. I never over drink. Because I drank too much that one time, I didn't say, "Okay now I had two drinks, next time I am going to have ten drinks." When it comes to eating, if someone is in bondage to food and they overeat just a little bit, they end up in an all-out binge because they will say to themselves, "Well now that I failed, I will just go ahead and eat the whole gallon of ice cream." It's against their rules, so they say, "I am a failure, I took a step backwards, and now I am going to go all the way back and eat the entire gallon." If you are not a sweets person, maybe it's the chips and queso at the Mexican restaurant.

I want you to say this to yourself over and over: If I am going to House B from House A and I stumble backwards 3 steps, I am not going to go all the way back to House A if my goal is house B. If I have three chips, I am not going to eat the entire bowl if my goal is to beat the bondage of food.

My mom owns a Christian counseling practice. One time I called her and I was really stressed because had one of the worst days ever at work. I found out that one of my managers was having an affair, and I was really upset. I also found out that another manager was lying to me about something else. I was overwhelmed at the idea of getting rid of two high level managers and didn't know if I should show grace or let them go. I had come home that day and taken my frustration out on food. My mom said to me "What would happen if you did fire them? Play the whole thing out in your mind." I said, "That would be a really horrible day." I just didn't know what to do. I felt like I was so stressed and she kept saying "Well what would happen?" over and over. I said, "I would be really upset, I really like them." She said, "Yea, that would be a horrible day for you wouldn't it?" I said, "Yes, it would be horrible and I have no idea how I would make it through." She said, "But you would get through it right?" And I said, "Yea, God would get me through it." As soon as I started talking out loud about it, I felt like I wasn't as fearful. I told her how I had come home that day and eaten all this comfort food out of my pantry. She said "Did you eating that food help you in any way to feel comforted? Did it help you with making a decision about what you needed to do? Did it make you feel better?" It made me feel better for only the four minutes that I was actually eating the food. Then it made me feel worse because those foods didn't make me feel good. They made me feel fat and guilty. I know that will be the outcome and I need to give myself a pep talk before I raid the pantry.

It's kind of like the ad where he said, "I should have had a V8". He's eating all this different food and then after the fact, he thinks "Rats, I should have had the V8 instead!" All of the people who say "I should have," "I need to," or "I ought to," are speaking are stress words. Instead, say preference words to calm you down such as "I'd like to" or "I'd prefer to." Just those words will calm you down. Until you are aware of what you are doing, you can't make the decision not to. Until you are more aware of what you are doing, you can't change. You learn and practice catching yourself before going to the damaging behavior. Become aware of what your triggers are that get you into that negative thinking.

For me, I have to say, "Okay, when I am stressed, I usually want to go to the pantry, so when I go home, I am not going to walk into the kitchen. I am going to walk right upstairs and draw a bath. Or I am going to walk upstairs, change my clothes, and go for a walk."

#2 Take Personal Responsibility

To break the bondage, you have to accept your share of responsibility for the problem. Understand this is not your husband's or your children's problem. Constantly blaming other people for why this is an issue in your life is counterproductive. Sometimes, I blame my husband because I wouldn't eat dinner if not for him. I'm never really hungry at night and I could fast during that time, but my husband wants a huge meal and sometimes I finish my son's plate. If he ate his own food, I wouldn't be finishing it. See the blame game? It's stupid, right? You need to fully take responsibility and say **"I take personal responsibility for allowing myself to be addicted to _____."**

You can't play the blame game.

#3 Share the Problem

1 John 1:9 (NIV)
⁹ If we confess our sins, he is faithful and just and will forgive us our sins and purify us from all unrighteousness.

Confess your sins to others you trust. Make a vow to change.

If you are carrying guilt, by talking about it, you are releasing it. You become more accountable for your sin by facing the problem. You have to name

---

your sin, label it, and identify it. If you aren't aware of the problem, you can't solve the problem. Think about it. With Alcoholics Anonymous, the first thing they do in each meeting is say "Hi I am Suzie, and I am an Alcoholic." They are claiming and labeling their sin before they move forward with the meeting.

#4 Get Rid of the Negative Influences.

If you have friends that are obviously drinking too much or friends that are doing drugs, you're not going to be able to hang out with those people and break free. You need to get rid of those influences in your life. If you have certain friends that think it's fun to overeat and encourage you to overeat, then they're people you have to step away from for the time being.

#5 Flee Temptation

I have a good friend who recently got divorced and is dating a new girl. Someone gave him tickets to go to a baseball game in Washington D.C., and it was too expensive for him to get two hotel rooms so they shared one room and slept in separate beds. He told me that nothing inappropriate happened, but looking back, he said that he knew it would have been more wise to spend the money for two separate rooms. Instead of fleeing temptation, he was setting himself up for temptation, and relying solely on his own willpower.

For me, my temptation is food. If I am feeling really stressed and I come home from work, I can't hang out in the kitchen. I have to flee that area by going for a walk or taking a bath. I am not going to go to a buffet with friends. If I am already feeling vulnerable, it doesn't make sense for me to hang out with temptation, I have to flee it.

If you struggle with pornography, you have to make really decisive actions to flee temptation. If you go to a hotel, you have to set up controls so that adult channels aren't available to you. Call your cable company to put the block on! There are apps and programs that block the porn from your phone, or even send a list of sites that you visit to the accountability partner of your choice. If you're going to a Bachelor party and your friends want to go seem some dancers, first of all, you need new friends! Second of all, tell them you will join them for dinner and then call it a night. Like my friend with the hotel room in D.C., you can't rely on your will power! You have to make really conscious, decisive actions to flee temptation.

#6 Quote God's Word

When Jesus was faced with temptation, he found a verse of Scripture that applied to that specific temptation and then He quoted it to Himself and the Devil. That is really powerful! He kept saying "it is written" over and over again. As followers of Christ in our fight against temptation, we often use the wrong weapons! We try to defeat this with our own power and our own flesh. A lot of people wonder if there really is a devil, but the Bible is very clear that there is. Some of my friends who aren't mature Christians may not think there is a devil, but this is what you can do to overcome your daily temptation every time.

You can use different verses for different problems.

- If you have a problem with lust use:

1 Thessalonians 4:3 (NIV)

³ It is God's will that you should be sanctified: that you should avoid sexual immorality;

1 Thessalonians 4:7 (NIV)

⁷ For God did not call us to be impure, but to live a holy life.

- If you're struggling with fear, use:

Isaiah 43:1-2 (NIV)

⁴³ But now, this is what the Lord says—

he who created you, Jacob,

he who formed you, Israel:

"Do not fear, for I have redeemed you;

I have summoned you by name; you are mine.

² When you pass through the waters,

I will be with you;

and when you pass through the rivers,

they will not sweep over you.

When you walk through the fire,

you will not be burned;

the flames will not set you ablaze.

- If you have a problem with gossip, use:

Ephesians 4:29 (NIV)

[29] Do not let any unwholesome talk come out of your mouths, but only what is helpful for building others up according to their needs, that it may benefit those who listen.

- If your problem is laziness, use:

Colossians 3:23-24 (NIV)

[23] Whatever you do, work at it with all your heart, as working for the Lord, not for human masters, [24] since you know that you will receive an inheritance from the Lord as a reward. It is the Lord Christ you are serving.

- For overeating, use:

Psalm 81:10 (NIV)

[10] I am the Lord your God,

who brought you up out of Egypt.

Open wide your mouth and I will fill it.

#7 Fast with Intensity

In order for you to have a meaningful fast, you can't just withhold food, but you have to agonize in prayer. Fasting communicates to everyone, including God, the seriousness of this issue.

> **This is your affirmation, "I believe that there is no earthly temptation that can enslave me but that God has a way of escape for me." (1 Corinthians 10:13, NIV)**

#8 Make the Commitment.

I am going to start my fast on _____ and end my fast on _____.

Isaiah 58:6 (NIV)

6 "Is not this the kind of fasting I have chosen:

to loose the chains of injustice

and untie the cords of the yoke,

to set the oppressed free

and break every yoke?

(Scriptural Basis)

This is when I am going to start my fast, this is when I am going to end my fast, and these are the people I am going to bring with me to the fast. If you can get a small group of people to fast with you, it is such a powerful thing. Fast and specifically pray for whatever is going on in each other's lives. You can all use this fast to pray about different people together and offer each other support throughout the fast.

The people following Ezra fasted because they were scared. They wanted safety for themselves and for their children. The bigger the problem, the more likely people will fast with intensity and really pray.

Ezra 8:21 (NIV)

[21] There, by the Ahava Canal, I proclaimed a fast, so that we might humble ourselves before our God and ask him for a safe journey for us and our children, with all our possessions.

CLOSING THOUGHTS

A lot of times, people fast about a problem for one day and if nothing changes they decide that they're not healed. You have to fast **repeatedly** until you get a breakthrough. Sometimes, you can pray and get an answer right away, but sometimes you have to keep fasting and praying over and over until you get your breakthrough.

One time I was visiting my family in San Francisco and the roads there are so windy! There were some streets that are so skinny, you don't think you can get through. You are literally like "There is no way I can get through this". There is a sign on one of the roads that says "Oh yes, you can!" Every time I am in a tough place with fasting, I think to myself "Oh, yes you can!" People say I can't fast! And I want you to think to yourself, "Oh yes, I can!"

Printed in the United States
By Bookmasters